Essential Oils:

A Beginner's Guide to Essential Oils. 200+ Essential Oils Recipes & Tips - Aromatherapy Natural Homemade Remedies to Improve Your Skin, Health, Lose Weight, Overcome Anxiety, Depression, & Stress!

Kevin Gise © 2017

Disclaimer:

Introduction

First off, thanks for grabbing my book "Essential Oils: A Beginner's Guide to Essential Oils. 200+ Essential Oils Recipes & Tips - Aromatherapy Natural Homemade Remedies to Improve Your Skin, Health, Lose Weight, Overcome Anxiety, Depression, & Stress!" By picking up this book you've shown that you're serious about learning all the possibilities afforded to us when using essential oils in our everyday lives.

This book will show you what you need in order to get started using essential oils. I'll be discussing the kinds of essential oils and all of their great benefits. I'll also be going over a bunch of carrier oils used to help create essential oil recipes and all the different ways these oils can be used to improve your life. I hope you enjoy essential oils the same way I have over the years. It's had a big impact on the lives of my friends and family.

Throughout this book, I'll be going over different recipes and tips I use. I've also included answers to some of the frequently asked questions I hear from newbies. You don't need to have any prior experience with essential oils in order for this book to benefit you.

I'm ready to get started. Let's begin!

Chapter One: A Beginner's Guide to Essential Oils

A Beginner's Guide to Essential Oils

An essential oil is a kind of liquid that is generally distilled (usually by steam or water) from leaves, stems, flower, bark, roots and other elements of a plant. Even though referred to as an oil, they do not give off an oily feeling. Many essential oils are actually clear, while some like orange, patchouli, and lemongrass are yellow or amber in color.

Essential oils are so wonderful because they contain the pure essence of the plant it's derived from. Since essential oils come highly concentrated, a tiny bit will go a long way. Many people confuse essential oils with fragrance oils or perfume. They are not the same. While essential oils are derived from the actual plant, perfumes and fragrance oils are created artificially and therefore may contain artificial ingredients. Perfumes and fragrance oils do not contain any of the therapeutic benefits associated with essential oils.

The aroma and chemical composition of essential oils can provide physical therapeutic benefits along with valuable psychological benefits. These benefits are normally achieved through the application of the oil to your skin or by inhalation.

Essential oils have been around for thousands of years. Many cultures have you used them to treat and alleviate illnesses throughout history. Every major civilization from the ancient Egyptians onward has harnessed the power of essential oils to improve the life of its people. Essential oils were so important that two of the three gifts said to be given to Jesus were myrrh and frankincense, both forms of powerful essential oils.

Many essential oils are often used by diluting them using a carrier oil and then applying the blend to your skin for absorption. A few examples of carrier oils are apricot kernel oil, sweet almond oil, and grapeseed oil.

Carefully inhaling certain essential oils can also have a therapeutic benefit. As oil molecules enter into the lungs they get absorbed into your bloodstream.

Essential oils normally get sold in tiny individual bottles. They can vary a great deal in both price and quality. Some of the factors that will affect the price and quality of your oil will include the plant's rarity, the standards of the people distilling the oil, the country, and climate where the oil comes from, and how much oil gets produced per plant.

When purchasing essential oils you can get either individual oils or blends of several oils. The advantage of purchasing blends is that it can save you time and money having to buy each individual oil and mixing them. The main disadvantage is that since you're not mixing it personally, you have no control over the blend and you can't reliably mix the blend you've purchased with any other oils.

Extraction Process

Essential oils are extracted from nature using a few different processes that I will discuss in this section.

Distillation

The majority of essential oils are obtained through this process. Raw plant materials such as roots, seeds, fruit peels, woods, and leaves are placed inside a distillation device. The water in the device containing the plant parts is then heated and the steam is passed through the device eventually vaporizing all the volatile compounds which are collected in a receiving vessel. This process will normally take several hours from start to finish. Some essential oils obtained using this process include lemon, lavender, and clary sage.

There are different forms of distillation from the one I mentioned above. Some of these are water distillation, steam distillation, and hydro-diffusion.

Expression

This process involves obtaining the essential oil through mechanical extraction. It is often referred to as cold pressing. The process was more popular before distillation was invented. It involves getting the essential oil from citrus peels. This method works on citrus essential oils only and was often done by hand. The peels contain a good amount of essential oil in them.

First, the peel or rind would be soaked in warm water, then a sponge would be used to press on the peel or rind. This would break up the protective layer of the peel and soak up the essential oil. Once that was completed, the sponge would be pressed over some form of container to collect the essential oil. Once pressed into the container, it would be left to stand so the oil had time to separate from the juice water. The final step would then involve siphoning the essential oil from the container. More modern methods of expression include the use of centrifuges and other modern machinery.

Solvent Extraction

This process involves extracting essential oils from plant parts containing small amounts of oil. For example, extracting essential oils from flowers is notoriously difficult due to the small amount of essential oil they contain. Therefore a solvent, such as hexane, is used to get the essential oil. These finished products are also referred to as absolutes, which I discussed in the last section.

Essential Oils Methods

Adding essential oils to your life can be fun, easy, and beneficial to your health. In this section, I'll be going over some of the ways you can get started. Each of these different methods provides their own set of benefits and safety concerns. Always be sure to follow all applicable safety precautions and pay attention to how certain oils are to be used or not used in specific situations. Don't forget that essential oils are powerful and therefore need to be used with some caution. It's also important to keep in mind that essential oils are also flammable so keep them away from open flames or sparks.

Bath

Add the amount of essential oil called for in your recipe to your carrier oil. Mix it together and add your blend to your running water in the bath. Be sure to mix it again before entering the tub. Always be sure to read any safety information on the oils you end up using.

Aromatherapy Massage

Add the amount of essential oil called for in your recipe to your carrier oil and massage the mixture on your partner or yourself. Always be sure to keep these blends away from your genitals, eyes, and mouth. Never apply essential oils directly to your skin without diluting the oil first. Always be sure to read any safety information on the oils you end up using.

Insect Repellent

Add the amount of essential oil called for in your recipe to your cotton balls or tissues and place them near your windows and doors to repel any insects. There are a ton of wonderful oils that act as a repellent for insects. These include peppermint, lavender, and my personal favorite citronella. During the summer, when I'm having guests over, I have posts surrounding my yard which I use citronella oil on. This helps to repel any insects from bothering us. Always be sure to read any safety information on the essential oils you end up using.

General Household Cleaning

Add the amount of essential oil called for in your recipe to your wash, trash can, drain, laundry, tissue, or vacuum bag filter. There are a million ways to incorporate essential oils into your household on a daily basis. Always be sure to read any safety information on the oils you end up using.

Pet Care

Add the amount of essential oil called for in your recipe to your carrier oil. Apply to your pets as laid out in the directions of whatever recipe you're using. Always be sure to read any safety information on the oils you end up using. Be very careful when using essential oils on your pets. I recommend not trying this until you've gained some experience working with them.

Normal Inhalation

Place approximately 3 to 4 drops of your essential oil on your tissue. Place your tissue near your nose area and deeply inhale. When first trying out an oil, only use a single drop to ensure that you're not sensitive or allergic to that type of essential oil. Always be sure to read any safety information on the oils you end up using.

Room Freshening

Add the amount of essential oil called for in your recipe to 2 cups of boiling water that's been placed in a bowl. Don't inhale into the bowl, instead, let the steam carry the oil throughout the room. Some people use this method, while many stick to scent rings or diffusers. I personally have a diffuser in every room of my home. Always be sure to read any safety information on the oils you end up using.

Steam Inhalation

Boil 2 cups of water. Pour your water into your bowl and add approximately 3 to 7 drops of essential oil to your water. You may want to consider using fewer drops if you're dealing with an oil that can cause irritation to your mucous membranes. For example, cinnamon, rosemary, thyme eucalyptus, and pine.

Place your nose approximately 12 inches away from your bowl and deeply inhale. Be sure not to inhale the steam on a constant basis. If you start to feel any kind of discomfort, stop right away. Steam inhalation is great for dealing with influenza and colds. Use of relaxing or energizing essential oils can also make this particular method useful. Keep your eyes closed when inhaling the steam. Always be sure to read any safety information on the oils you end up using.

Other Uses

Besides the methods listed above, essential oils can be made into facial toners, lotions, soaps, perfumes, shampoos, and other types of natural products. Essential oils are extremely versatile in the ways they can be used to benefit us in our daily lives. In this book alone I go over more than 350 essential oil recipes you can use to help benefit you, your pets, or your home.

Aromatherapy Basics

Aromatherapy is, in essence, the practice of using different varieties of volatile plant oils, including essential oils, for our physical, spiritual, emotional, and mental well-being.

In addition to using essential oils, aromatherapy also encourages the use of other types of complementary naturally found ingredients including hydrosol, sugars, sea salts, clay, herbs, milk powders, mud, cold pressed vegetable oils, and jojoba (a type of liquid wax).

Aromatherapy frowns up the use of any kind of synthetic ingredients being used. Always be careful when purchasing products that are marketed with the word aromatherapy on their labeling or packaging. This word is not regulated in the US and many products out there on the market contain ingredients that are synthetic. These products should be avoided. That's why it's always important to read the labels before you buy.

The same can be said for items labeled essential oils or natural ingredients. Those labels can be misleading and may contain synthetic ingredients along with the oils or natural ingredients they are claiming to be made with. Good sellers should always be happy to provide you with a list of the ingredients in their essential oils or other products. That's why I suggest only purchasing your essential oils and supplies through reputable companies. In the resource section, I give a bunch of reputable places I use to purchase my essential oils.

Topical Application Essential Oils Benefits

Essential oils that are topically applied to your skin get absorbed into your bloodstream. The constituents of an essential oil can aid in areas like beauty, health, and hygiene. Since essential oils are incredibly concentrated and powerful, they shouldn't be applied topically to your skin in their undiluted form.

To apply an essential oil to your skin, one should dilute the essential oil using a carrier oil. A few examples of carrier oils include grapeseed oil, sweet almond oil, and apricot kernel oil. I'll touch on a few more different kinds of carrier oil in the next chapter.

Inhaling Essential Oils Benefits

Essential oils that are inhaled into your lungs can offer both physical and psychological benefits. The aroma of your essential oil stimulates your brain to trigger a specific reaction, but when it is inhaled into your lungs, the natural constituents can supply a wonderful therapeutic benefit. For example, diffusing eucalyptus oil can help you ease congestion. Always be sure to use your essential oils correctly. Not doing so could have serious repercussions and side effects.

Other Essential Oil Benefits

In addition to the emotional, spiritual, mental, and therapeutic benefits of essential oils, they can be used in a variety of other applications. Essential oils can be used in natural pesticides and insect repellent, household cleaners, and pet care.

Essential Oil Blends

A big upside of essential oils is that they can be mixed and matched to form new complex blends and aromas. In a later chapter, I'll go over 350+ recipes you can make on your own for a variety of different applications. Oftentimes, essential oils that are blended together can have a greater effect than if you had them working independently.

You should always be careful when blending together essential oils. When you're first starting out I would steer clear of any of the oils I mention as hazardous in the next chapter. I would also hold off on using them around children, pets, or pregnant women until you have much more experience working with them. It's always a good idea to find a good aromatherapist in your area and have them help you with any blends or recipes that can cause serious side effects if done improperly.

Diffusers Types

I will often get asked what kinds of diffusers are best and what are the differences between the different types of diffusers. Unfortunately, there's no one right answer to this question. A lot of this comes down to personal preference or the specific situation you're using the diffuser for. In this section, I'll discuss the four different categories of available diffusers. Each type of these diffusers puts your essential oils into the air. Each one has its own set of benefits to consider. I use everything but heat diffusers. I don't like to heat up my essential oils but that's just a personal preference.

<u>Heat Diffusers</u>

These are similar to the evaporative diffusers, however, they use heat instead of air blowing to accomplish the diffusion. While some types of heat diffusers will use a higher level of heat to produce a stronger smell, the top heat diffusers only use a lower level of heat to produce a more subtle and subdued aroma. The level of heat you're using is very important. The higher the heat the more you can alter the chemical properties of your essential oils.

These types of diffusers share the same issues as the evaporative diffusers. They don't get the whole essential oil at once. The good thing about these diffusers is they are completely silent and cost effective to use. They do a good job of putting your oil's aroma into your room.

Evaporative Diffusers

These diffusers are pretty simplistic in the way they operate. You have a fan that blows air from your room through a filter or pad that contains essential oils dropped on it. The air that is blowing through your pad causes your oils to evaporate at a quicker rate than normal, while the air containing your evaporated oil is being blown into your room.

This type of diffuser is ideal for getting your oil scent into your room. However, due to the way it evaporates you don't get the whole essential oil all at once. Instead, you get the lighter components in the oil at the start of the process and the heavier components near the end of the process. What this means is that the therapeutic properties of the oil may be diminished thereby lessening the effects.

Overall, this is a good form of diffusion that quietly diffuses your aroma throughout an entire room. They make a wide variety of these diffusers. Everything from battery operated versions to diffuser jewelry versions which you can wear.

Humidifying / Ultrasonic Diffusers

Similar to nebulizing diffusers, ultrasonic diffusers will also create a fine mist. However, the method it uses to accomplish this is very different. With an ultrasonic diffuser your utilizing different electronic frequencies to make a small-sized disk under the surface of a liquid, like water, to begin vibrating at an extremely fast rate. These ultrasonic vibrations will then break your essential oils down into tiny micro-sized particles, dispersing your oil in the form of a fine mist. These smaller particles are much more easily absorbed by your lungs for a better therapeutic effect on your mind, spirit, and body.

While transforming water or liquids into a vapor will normally require a lot of heat, the transformation of your liquids into a vapor occurs through an adiabatic process. This means the means the liquids changed states without using any type of heat energy.

This kind of diffusion will make a nice mist that will humidify the air and gives off the sound of water trickling, although only a tiny amount of your mist is actually your essential oil and it will depend completely on the room's air current to actually disperse your mist through the entire room. This makes this type of diffuser ideal for people who only want a small amount of essential oil to be diffused into their room.

Nebulizing Diffusers

A nebulizer basically works in the same fashion a perfume atomizer does. A small jet of air blowing across a small-sized tube creates a type of vacuum that actually pulls your liquid at the bottom of your tube up to the top of your tube. The air that is flowing across the surface of your oil at the top of your tube blows your oil away in a mist or fine spray. When used with a consistent air supply source, this kind of diffusion will put a lot of oil in the air quickly.

Since this kind of diffusion is working to put your whole oil out into the air in tiny droplet form, it's often thought to be the best kind of diffusion for the therapeutic use of your essential oils. Since these nebulizing diffusers are working to quickly saturate the air with your essential oil, they will normally run at a higher level of sound and will also use your essential oil at a much higher rate than the other kinds of diffusers. When using these diffusers it's a good idea to run them on a timer so that there only running for approximately 15 minutes every hour. This will allow you to conserve your essential oil and cut down on your costs. It will also allow your olfactory system some time to process the oils that you've received and allow you to recover before getting more.

Essential Oils Uses

Essential oils are so popular because they offer solutions to so many different problems people face in their day to day lives. This versatility is virtually unmatched by any other set of products I can think of. In this section, I'm going to go over some of the many reasons one can use essential oils.

Congestion, Colds, & Flu

Don't like taking pills and other forms of doctor prescribed medication? Want something natural to help you get rid of that cold or your cough? If so, then you'll want to check out some of the recipes I have that focus in treating colds, flu, & congestion using a variety of essential oils. I also include recipes to help boost your immune system so you never fall ill in the first place.

Common Ailments, Pains, & Aches

Essential oils are wonderful for treating everything from minor aches and pulled muscles, to sores, cuts, and burns. If there's something wrong with your body there's more than likely a combination of essential oils that can help ease your discomfort and quicken the healing process.

Cleaning Products

If you don't want to clean your home using products filled with harmful chemicals then you're going to love all the cleaning recipes I've included later on in this book. I try and use as many of these as I can in my own home. Not only are they a healthier alternative to store bout solutions they're also effective. It's hard to beat a combination like that.

Mental Clarity & Emotional Support

Essential oils are often used to help treat conditions like depression. Essential oils can stimulate the limbic system in our brain. They can be used for all different types of emotional issues ranging from anger and abandonment issues to grief, worthlessness, and fear of failure. Essential oils are also great for helping us focus and achieve mental clarity. Back in college, I used to use essential oils whenever I had to study for an exam. I'm naturally unfocused, meaning I could always use the extra boost my essential oils provided me with.

Energy & Mood

Not only can essential oils keep us relaxed they can also be used to give us a shot of much-needed energy. Not only that but certain essential oils can directly affect a person's mood and outlook on life. I love using my oils whenever I'm feeling a little down or lazier than usual. I find they do an excellent job of lifting my spirits and getting my engine going. I've included many of my favorite recipes in a later chapter of this book.

Relationships & Love

Looking for love in your life? Want to attract someone? Aroma plays a big part in who we desire and who we don't. I've included a few aphrodisiacs to help you find that special someone in your life.

Room Freshener

Essential oils can be used to make your home smell fresh and inviting. I've included a bunch of recipes perfect for all types of occasions and seasons.

Pet Care

Essential oils can be great for your pets. I've included a bunch of different recipes you can use to help improve the life of your pet. I suggest not trying these on your pets before you've got some experience handling essential oils. Personally, I waited a long time before ever using an essential oil on them. I tend to err on the side of caution but the safety of my pet is always my utmost concern.

Relaxation

Essential oils are excellent for helping one center themselves and find a deeper sense of peace and relaxation. Different recipes and aromas have a way of triggering our mind to slow down and remove any anxiety or stress that may be negatively affecting us.

Weight Loss

If you want to drop a few pounds then essential oils like grapefruit oil, ginger oil, and cinnamon oil will aid you in the process. I've included recipes for everything from cellulite removers and appetite suppressors to metabolism boosters and weight loss remedies.

Hair Care & Skin

Essential oils can treat everything from a mild case of acne to a severe form of eczema. Essential oils can also protect your lips, hands, feet, and hair. In a later chapter, I'll be going over a bunch of different recipes to combat all forms of skin and hair care issues. Not only can essential oils help cure existing issues it can also help prevent issues in the future. It will make your skin and hair healthier than ever before.

Essential Oil Safety

Essential oils can be harmful if not handled appropriately. These are highly concentrated liquids and are very powerful even in small doses. This power means when used correctly they can be extremely beneficial. Unfortunately if used in an improper manner they can have dangerous side effects. Implementing essential oils into your lifestyle doesn't need to be a stressful or worrisome situation, but it's important that you learn about using these oils safely and in an appropriate manner. By treating the use of essential oils with caution and respect, you'll be on your way to safely benefit from all that these wonderful oils have to offer.

This section on safety is by no way a complete safety reference guide. Every oil has its own set of rules you'll want to abide by. Always be sure to research the oils you're using before actually using them. If you're ever in doubt I suggest consulting a trained aromatherapy practitioner or your doctor. It's always best to err on the side of caution. The last thing you want to do is cause more harm than good. The whole point of using essential oils is to improve your life.

Essential oils shouldn't ever be used on your skin undiluted While an experienced user or trained professional may make exceptions to this rule on occasion, someone newer to essential oils should never make that attempt on their own. Many times you'll see people say that tea tree oil and lavender oil can be used undiluted. I suggest not trying this as a certain percentage of people will still suffer from a severe reaction to the undiluted oil. It's better to be safe and **NEVER** use any type of essential oil undiluted.

When you apply an essential oil for the first time on your skin, I suggest using a skin patch test on a tiny area of your skin to make sure you're not allergic or sensitive to the oil. Everyone is different. Certain oils will affect people in different ways. No one's body chemistry is exactly the same. It's always best to test before jumping in.

Essential oils aren't highly regulated. This means knowing exactly what is in each bottle is hard to know. This makes buying only high-quality essential oils from known and respected companies very important. Don't go with a company that has no reputation or a bad reputation. You need to have confidence that you're getting what you paid for when buying your essential oils. I go over a few of the places I use and trust in a later chapter.

Another thing to be aware of is that some types of essential oils are what is known as phototoxic. What is that you ask? Well, this means these oils can cause inflammation, redness, burning, and irritation when they get exposed to any UVA rays. You'll see in a few of the recipes I've included that I mention not to go directly into the sunlight once you've applied it topically. This is because they contain phototoxic oils which can lead to one of the side effects above. Always be sure to check the side effects of essential oils before using them. You also want to check if they have any harmful interactions when mixed with other specific oils or drugs.

There are many types of essential oils that need to be avoided by certain groups of people. For instance, children and pregnant women have certain oils they should not be using. Also, people suffering from certain health conditions like epilepsy and asthma will need to steer clear of certain essential oils. Don't forget to check an essential oils safety information before using it.

Many people underestimate the strength of essential oils. This is one of those things where less is definitely more. When using these oils you want to always use the least amount that will get the job you're trying to accomplish done. If a recipe calls for 2 drops, only use 2 drops. These oils are very concentrated and using more than what is called for can have unintended side effects or just be wasteful.

Don't get suckered in by people or businesses telling you to use as much of their products in one sitting as you'd like. Those people are trying to improve their bottom line. They are not thinking about your overall well-being. The faster you go through your oils the quicker you'll need to reorder more. Essential oils are not inexpensive. Be mindful of this when using them. Your wallet will thank you.

Do not use any of the hazardous oils I'll go over later in this chapter. These oils can be dangerous and if used, should only be done so by an experienced aromatherapy practitioner. Even then I suggest avoiding these oils. There's no need to put your health or well-being at risk.

Always keep children away from your essential oils. Keep your oils stored in a safe and secure location within your home. Many oils have a pleasant smell and unsuspecting children will think they are safe to ingest or use in a large amount, undiluted on their skin. Treat your essential oils like they were prescription medicine. They can be very dangerous in the hands of those not educated on how to use them.

When first starting out never take essential oils internally without consulting an expert or physician first. This may change once you've gained enough experience but it's not worth the risk when you don't fully grasp everything involved. People new to essential oils will often get the dosage or recipe wrong and end up harming themselves. Don't let this be you!

Don't forget that essential oils are very flammable. Always keep them away from open flames and other fire hazards. Be diligent with this. I've heard a few horror stories over the years. It's a simple precaution to take but one with steep consequences if ignored.

Six Essential Oils Safety Factors

Most of this I discussed above but here are six factors that can influence how safe the essential oils we use are. Knowing these will allow you to make smarter decisions when choosing the essential oils you want to incorporate into your daily life.

1. Application Method

Essential oils can be used in a variety of ways. They can be applied topically, diffused, inhaled, and ingested. Each one of these methods has their own set of safety issues to contend with. Ingestion can be the most dangerous. Ingesting the wrong type or amount of oil can lead to coma and even death. When applying topically one must make sure that they are not sensitive or allergic to the oil in question. You'll also want to check the phototoxicity of an oil and whether it has any harmful interactions when mixed with other oils or medications. Topically applied oil can cause irritation and even burns when not used correctly. Diffusion and inhalation have the lowest risks associated with them. In more extreme cases you may begin to get headaches, lethargy, vertigo, and nausea when using them incorrectly.

2. Quality

The less pure an essential oil the more likely you'll have an adverse response to it. Always try and use the purest essential oils you can find. The more authentic the better off you'll be.

3. Dosage

Always be sure to use the right amount of oil. Never use more than what is called for. Doing so will only increase the level of danger. Always dilute your oil when using topically. Blending oils and carrier oils can mitigate the negative effects they may have otherwise.

4. Skin Integrity

Damaged, inflamed, or diseased skin is more permeable to essential oils and can be much more sensitive to a dermal reaction. It's potentially very dangerous to put any undiluted essential oils on your damaged, inflamed, or diseased skin. Under that kind of circumstance, one's skin condition may become worse, and a larger amount of the oil will be absorbed than is normal. The rate of sensitization reactions will also rise on damaged, inflamed, and diseased skin.

5. Chemical Composition

Essential oils rich in aldehydes and phenols may at times cause bad skin reactions. Essential oils that are rich in that kind of constituents should always be diluted prior to any application on the skin. Always be aware of the chemical composition of the oils you choose to use.

6. Health & Age

Infants and younger children are much more sensitive to the potency of various essential oils than adults are. The same can be said for elderly users, pregnant women, and people suffering from certain medical conditions. Always know what types of oils are appropriate for the people using them. Just because it's safe for you doesn't mean that applies to everyone else.

Chapter Two: Essential Oils Frequently Asked Questions

Essential Oils Frequently Asked Questions

In this chapter, I will go discuss some of the common questions I come across the most when talking about essential oils. I hope you're able to find sufficient answers to whatever remaining questions you have.

1. How Often Should I Use Essential Oils?

I hear this one a lot and there's no one right answer. Personally, I suggest using essential oils on a needed basis. By doing this you're preventing your body from becoming too accustomed to your oils, negating the beneficial effects. For essential oils that you need to use on a normal basis, like those for sleep, I recommend alternating the types of calming oils you use.

2. How Do I Use My Essential Oils?

Essential oils can be used in a variety of different ways. Here are the main ones:

Aromatically – Diffusing essential oils in the air surrounding you is a nice way to reap all the benefits of your essential oils. I use diffusers in each room of my house so I can use my oils whenever and wherever I want to.

Topically – Many types of essential oils are meant to be applied directly on your skin, diluting them using a carrier oil.

Internally - A few higher quality essential oils are safe to be ingested internally.

3. What Things Should I Keep An Eye Out For When Dealing With Essential Oils?

When using essential oils, you should use the highest quality oils you're able to afford.

Look for companies growing the plants they use in their oils without using pesticides. A certified organic company will always be my preference. You can find out if the company you're thinking of using meets those standards by either visiting their website or contacting them directly.

While some companies make essential oils that are pure enough to be ingested internally, many essential oils being made are diluted with a carrier oil or were derived from plants that were grown using pesticides. You wouldn't want to ingest those oils internally.

Seek out oils that have been tested for their purity before being sold. The purer the essential oil the better. I like oils without any additives in them, like carrier oils.

4. Can You Ingest Essential Oils?

You can ingest certain essential oils, however, I would suggest avoiding doing that. Be sure to vet a company that directs you to take their oils internally and be sure to follow their instructions exactly. If you have doubts, I'd suggest not taking them or contact the company directly for more information.

If an essential oil is safe to consume you can try taking them using these methods:

Under Your Tongue – Some essential oils, like digestive essential oil blends, are best when taken underneath your tongue. Start out with a single drop, see how you're feeling after a few minutes and take another drop if needed. Relief should occur pretty quickly.

Capsule – A lot of companies will sell empty capsules online or in your local health food store. Capsules are a great way of taking essential oils that would usually burn your mouth if you took them undiluted or in water.

In Water – Some essential oils, like lemon, wild orange, and peppermint are good in water. The typical dilution ratio is approximately 1 drop per every 4 ounces of water.

5. How Are Essential Oils Used With Children?

Some essential oils are toxic to kids if they are taken in a big enough dose. For example, a big dose of wintergreen or a small dose taken internally of melaleuca. It's important that you treat your essential oils like they are medication and store them out of the reach of your children. Teach your kids about how to use essential oils so if they do get into them they understand how to use them safely.

Whenever I use essential oils on the children I'm always sure to dilute them in either a tub of bathwater or carrier oil. I also try and apply the oils to the bottoms of their feet. The reason behind this is because while the oil still enters the bloodstream quickly, the tougher skin on the bottom of feet isn't prone to getting irritated like most other parts of the body are.

Another tip is to watch over them while they learn to apply the oils themselves. I dilute the oil for them first while they watch but I like to let them apply it so that they can learn to do it for themselves when they are older.

6. What Is A Carrier Oil?

This is a type of oil that you use as a base in order to dilute other types of essential oils before you apply them to your skin. Diluting essential oils is a smart idea whenever using them.

7. What Kinds Of Essential Oils Are Safe For Women Who Are Pregnant?

Using essential oils while pregnant requires a little caution. For instance, be careful of what you're using during the first weeks of your pregnancy as this is a rapid time of development for your baby. I've included oils to avoid during pregnancy, but you should monitor yourself and how much oil you're using even if they aren't on this list.

Dilute your oils while pregnant. Don't apply an oil directly to your skin before doing so. Stick with aromatherapy whenever it's possible. Diffusing oils aromatically is a safer way to use your essential oils while pregnant. The majority of problems pregnant women have using essential oils during pregnancy arise from topical and internal use.

Essential Oils To Avoid During Pregnancy:

Birch

Aniseed

Camphor

Basil

Cinnamon Bark

Cassia

Clary Sage

Hyssop

Mugwort

Lemongrass

Parsley Leaf or Seed

Rosemary

Pennyroyal

Tansy

Sage

Tarragon

Thyme

Thuja

Vetiver

Wintergreen

White Fir

Wormwood

8. Are Essential Oils Allowed When Breastfeeding?

Yes. Here is a list of essential oils that are safe to use when breastfeeding.

Ylang Ylang

Lemon

Clary Sage

Geranium

Bergamot

Lavender

Grapefruit

Patchouli

Wild Orange

Sandalwood

Peppermint (Small Amounts)

Roman Chamomile

9. What Amount Of Essential Oils Should One Be Using?

A small amount can go a long way. Work up from one drop unless using a recipe that recommends otherwise.

10. What Kinds Of Precautions Are Needed When Using Essential Oils?

Although essential oils are natural, they are extremely potent. I advise using precaution when using them. Here are a few things to do when dealing with your essential oils.

1. Use higher quality oils whenever possible. The higher the quality the purer they usually are.

2. Keep away from your eyes.

3. If you doubt the strength of your oil dilute it.

4. Test the oils on your skin before using them topically. Make sure you don't have a negative reaction before applying the oil more liberally.

5. See how your body reacts. If something feels wrong, stop using that essential oil immediately.

6. If you have a negative reaction stop using that type of oil.

11. What Kinds Of Items Are Needed To Use Essential Oils Correctly?

Here are a few items you may find helpful having right from the start.

Bottles

Diffusers

Droppers

Carrier Oil

Cotton Balls

Reference Guide

12. How Do You Determine The Quality Of Your Essential Oil?

There are a bunch of variables that will come into play when determining the quality of your essential oil. Here are a few of the things that can affect the quality.

1. Rainfall amount.

2. Climate and altitude where it was originally grown.

3. Soil quality.

4. Harvesting methods.

5. The time that has passed between being harvested and being distilled.

6. Storage methods before being distilled.

7. The reputation of the company selling the oil. Certain companies are known for producing high-grade essential oils, while other less reputable companies may try blending pure essential oils with lower quality oils. Some of these less than reputable companies may also try and add synthetic constituents to their oil in an attempt to "improve" the low quality.

13. How Long Can Essential Oils Last?

Will essential oils last "forever". Unfortunately, the answer to that is no. Essential oils tend to be volatile, the more you open the bottle they are stored in the quicker all the constituents in your oil will start to evaporate. The shelf life of your essential oils will depend on the kind of oil and the manner in which it is stored. Here are some tips to help you improve the shelf life of your essential oils.

1. Always tightly close the lid after use.

2. Store away from the light. I keep my oils in a storage cabinet.

3. Keep cool. I know many people who refrigerate their oils in small fridges. Don't mix them in with any items you'll be ingesting.

Most citrus oils have a shelf life of between 1 year and 3 years, while woodsy oils can last for around a decade. If your oil ever begins to get thick, smell differently, or appear cloudy it's time to discard it. Better safe than sorry.

Chapter Three: 50+ Essential Oils Tricks & Tips

50+ Essential Oils Tricks & Tips

In this chapter, I'll be giving you 50+ tricks and tips I've come across during my time using essential oils. Some of these you may know already but I find a good amount of them are new to the majority of people. I hope they are able to help you out the same way they've helped me.

1. Keep your essential oils clear of any light, dampness, heat, and electromagnetic frequencies (TV's, microwaves).

2. Essential oils are extremely flammable. Be careful to avoid any sparks, open flames, and electricity to avoid fire hazards.

3. Essential oils are able to help renew our dying cells. That's why they are so popular for skin care.

4. Place a couple of drops of your favorite essential oil onto a cotton ball and place it in a vacuum cleaner bag before vacuuming.

5. Never allow essential oils to get into your eyes. If it does immediately seek help. Avoid getting essential oils into your nose or ears.

6. Add a few drops to your cornstarch or baking soda, mix together and allow it to set for a few days. Sprinkle it over your carpets. Allow to set for around an hour and then vacuum.

7. If you dislike the smell of an essential oil do not use it for emotional benefits. It won't have the intended effect.

8. Essential oils are natural antioxidants.

9. Clary sage and bergamot oils help people withdrawing from eating, alcohol, and smoking addictions.

10. Lavender oil is great for reducing itching associated with bug bites and lessening migraine severity.

11. Maximize the long-term effectiveness of your essential oils by taking short breaks from using them. For example, I take a few days off from using them each week. Some people prefer to use them for a couple weeks and then take off for an entire week. Choose the method that works best for you.

12. Avoid strong sunlight or tanning beds after applying your essential oils, especially when using phototoxic oils.

13. Clove, thyme, and lemon essential oils are excellent natural disinfectants.

14. Make heating pads out of some rice and a large sock. Just add your rice to the sock and sew it shut. Scent with your essential oil and microwave to heat up when you have aches or pains.

15. Cinnamon, myrrh, and frankincense are all thought to be strong anti-cancer and anti-tumor essential oils.

16. Making an essential oil all purpose cleaner is a great way to incorporate essential oils into your daily life. Combine 1 part vinegar, 2 parts water, and 5 drops of your desired essential oil in a glass spray bottle.

17. Aloe Vera will help to deepen the penetration of essential oils into your tissues, muscles, and joints.

18. It takes essential oils 1 second via inhalation and 3 seconds via skin application to reach your limbic system and begin to kick in.

19. Avoid purchasing any essential oils that have rubber glass dropper tops. Essential oils are extremely concentrated and will turn rubber into a gum-like substance which will ruin your essential oil.

20. Adding a few drops of your essential oil to a new roll of toilet paper will keep your bathroom smelling pleasant.

21. Fill up your spray bottle with water and add in a couple drops of essential oil to use as an air freshener.

22. Adding essential oils to wood dryer balls is a great way to help fluff and separate your laundry naturally. These balls will break up static and keep your laundry smelling fresh. Perfect alternative to dryer sheets.

23. Keep the garbage can smelling fresh by dropping your cotton ball dabbed in essential oil to the bottom of a garbage can in order to minimize any odors.

24. Use essential oils on your jewelry. Diffuser bracelets and necklaces can easily be made at home or purchased from a retailer. They will normally last about a day before needing to add more oil.

25. When applying essential oils for aromatic effects apply the oils to the skin close to your nose. You can also add it to the back of your neck, nose, temples, wrists, or on your jewelry.

26. Peppermint oil has been known to help people adapt to new ideas easier.

27. Add 2 to 3 drops of your desired essential oil onto a dried log. Allow the essential oil to soak in and then place your log on the fire to diffuse.

28. Store your oils in a dark, cool place away from the light. I have multiple storage boxes so I can move my oils around whenever necessary.

29. Lavender oils and tea tree oils can be applied to your cuts, scrapes, or scratches for pain relief and healing properties.

30. Add a few drops of essential oil to your hair rinse (around 5 to 7 drops in a cup of water). Massage it in thoroughly.

31. Purchase your essential oils from a reputable company. I have used the Global Aromatherapy Business Directory to help me find products and have been happy with the results. Don't purchase essential oils from vendors you don't know. I see people buy essential oils at local fairs and craft shows with no knowledge of the quality of the essential oil being purchased.

32. Place a dab of your essential oil on some cotton balls and place them around your house in out of the way spots like closets and drawers.

33. Add 3 to 5 drops of your essential oil directly to your rinse water when your washing clothes.

34. When you change your air filters used in the HVAC, add a couple drops of your essential oils to help filter and freshen the air as it is circulated throughout your home.

35. Add a couple drops of essential oil to your old and worn Potpourri in order to inject it with new life.

36. Wax warmers are a cheap way to distribute essential oils. Fill up your bowl with coconut oil and add a few drops of your favorite essential oils. Once your warmer gets hot the essential oils will scent the air.

37. Add one drop of lavender oil to the inside of a mascara tube to help it last longer and promote longer and thicker lashes.

38. Frankincense oil can help decrease an allergic reaction within a few seconds.

39. Place a couple drops of your essential oil into the melted hot wax of a candle that is burning. A nice way to diffuse the essential oil.

40. Place a couple drops of your lavender oil onto your pillow in order to induce pleasant dreams.

41. Perfume oils are different from essential oils. Many people get the two confused. Perfume oils don't contain any of the therapeutic benefits that essential oils offer.

42. Place your essential oils on scent rings, light bulbs, and radiators. Be sure to avoid any electrical sockets or outlets.

43. Essential oils have viscosity levels that can differ from one another. When baking, don't drop your oil directly into your mix. Drop the amount called for on a spoon first and make sure you have the proper amount before adding. Essential oils are concentrated and powerful. You never want to add more than what is called for.

44. Diffuse essential oils in your tissue box in order to create scented tissues to help with stuffy nose problems. Open your box, add a couple drops onto your tissues and close it back up.

45. Compare oils with the same names. Some plants have common names like anise, lavender, and eucalyptus. You need to always check the Latin botanical names to properly tell them apart. For example, two essential oils may be listed as lavender oil but they come from completely different plants. Since they come from separate plants the aroma and properties of each essential oil may differ. The same may be said of the cost. Some essential oils are more expensive because they are made from plants that are rare and difficult to find.

46. Want to make a quick air freshener? Wood is porous so take wooden clothes pins and place a couple drops of essential oils on them. Clip them anywhere you want to freshen up the air. Perfect for air vents in cars. You can also place your essential oils on wooden jewelry and wear your oils that way. If you don't have wood you can also use leather.

47. Place a couple drops of your essential oil either directly into your shoes or try dabbing some onto a cotton ball and put a cotton ball into each of your shoes.

48. Cinnamon oil has been known to help a home sell quicker. If you want to list your property, try putting out a few diffusers with cinnamon oil before holding open houses.

49. To avoid any drug induced interactions or side effects be sure to consult your doctor before trying essential oils. This is important if you're on medications as certain essential oils can heighten their effects.

50. Pay attention to any safety precautions or warnings when dealing with essential oils. This is very important when dealing with woman who are pregnant and children.

51. Many forms of citrus essential oils will make your skin photosensitive.

52. Create your own personalized bath salts using Epsom salts and leftover bottles of your essential oils. The salts will absorb the trace amounts of the essential oils left in your bottles. Feel free to mix and match your scents. To use, add 2 to 4 tablespoons of your salts to any bath.

53. Create your own personalized perfume by adding 10 to 25 drops of your preferred essential oil to perfume alcohol or 1 ounce of vodka.

54. Only work with your essential oils in an area where you have a good source of ventilation. Overuse of essential oils can lead to headaches or even dizziness so always be sure to take a break outdoors and work near an open window whenever possible.

Chapter Four: Basic Carrier Oils & Essential Oils Guide

Carrier Oil Types

In this part, I'm going to discuss a list of the common carrier oils and what they do. This will give you a helpful reference for later on when you're trying to determine what types of oils to use for the purpose you're trying to achieve.

Carrier oils are a necessity if you plan on using essential oils for anything besides cleaning products. A carrier oil is just a liquid form of vegetable oil that is used to help dilute the highly concentrated essential oil you want to use.

Here are my preferred carrier oils and a little bit about each one.

Coconut Oil

Perfect for moisturizing the hair, lips, and skin. Has lubricating properties which make it an ideal choice for massage. This carrier oil is a little harder to handle than some of the others as it remains a solid when at room temperature. Has a fragrant aroma and is very stable with an oily feel to it. I don't use this kind of oil too much as I'm not a big fan of the aroma.

Jojoba Oil

This is an extremely useful carrier oil and one of my top choices. This kind of carrier oil is really a wax. It's very stable to use and comes with a longer shelf life. This kind of oil acts like a natural anti-inflammatory and is perfect for inflamed skin or in the use of massage. This kind of oil is suited for people who are prone to acne and have oily skin. This carrier oil absorbs nicely and has a distinct smell that I quite enjoy.

Borage Seed Oil

This is a good choice when trying to treat a skin condition such as acne. It is also known for its anti-inflammatory properties and is helpful at combating gout, arthritis, and clotting disorders. This carrier oil should be avoided by pregnant women and those suffering from liver conditions.

Marula Oil

This is an excellent oil known for its wonderful antioxidant properties. It's easy to work with and extremely stable. Does a good job of both healing and hydrating your skin at the same time. This kind of carrier oil is harvested from the nut located inside the Marula fruit out of Africa. This is a perfect kind of oil for hair, skincare, and other beauty regimens.

Fractionated Coconut Oil

This is simply coconut oil that's had the longer chain fatty acids removed from it. The difference between this and regular coconut oil is that it stays liquid when at room temperature, making it much easier to handle and use in applications with essential oil. It's a very stable oil with a long shelf life and it's affordable which makes it a nice option if you're on a budget.

People who enjoy all natural oils will want to stay away from this carrier oil as it has been tampered with chemically to remove parts of its natural compounds. This oil is naturally odorless and colorless. It doesn't have a greasy feeling which is something I like.

Sweet Almond Oil

My favorite carrier oil. This is a wonderful all-purpose carrier oil. It's cheap to buy and has a shelf life of about 1 year. This kind of oil absorbs quickly while leaving only a small hint of oil on the skin. I use this type of oil in a ton of recipes later on in this guide. Keep this carrier oil on hand.

Essential Oils Types

In this part, I'm going to discuss a bunch of common essential oils and what they are best known for. This will give you a helpful reference for later on when you're trying to determine what kinds of essential oils to use for the purpose you're trying to achieve.

Bay Oil

This has a spicy, fruity, medicinal aroma to it. This a warming oil that is perfect for the fall and winter months. This oil is ideal for helping heal muscle pulls and muscle strains. It's also known for stimulating circulation. Other reasons for using this oil include the treatment of dandruff, treating oily skin, and hair care.

This oil can inhibit blood clotting so always be careful to use the amount recommended.

Angelica Root Oil

This has a woody and peppery aroma to it. This oil is known to stimulate one's immune system, fight off infection, and eliminate toxins. This oil has often been used in combating anxiety, stress, and different forms of exhaustion. This oil is intense and is often blended with other oils instead of being used solely on its own. It has a very distinctive woodsy and peppery aroma to it.

This is a phototoxic oil and once applied should not be directly in any type of UV light. Could cause blistering and irritation to the skin if it's exposed.

Basil Oil

This has a sweet licorice aroma to it. This is a great oil to use when needing to focus or stimulate your mind. It has many antiviral and antibacterial properties which make it ideal when feeling under the weather with a cold. This type of oil is also popular for treating flatulence, exhaustion, gout, flu, insect bites, and coughs.

Should preferably be used only during the morning hours and daytime hours. This type of oil should only be used sparingly.

Anise Oil

This has a rich licorice aroma to it. This is a strong essential oil known for its use in treating many types of ailments such as colds, congestion, flu, coughing, muscle aches, and flatulence. This kind of oil is also said to stimulate menstruation and increase the production of breast milk.

This essential oil should be avoided in children under the age of 5 and pregnant women.

Caraway Seed Oil

This has a spicy, sweet, and fruity aroma to it. This oil is used more in fragrance blends than holistic ones. When used holistically it is often a part of blends, especially those that are geared towards men. It's a good expectorant that is sometimes used in diffuser blends to help combat bronchitis and colds. This type of oil is also used as an energy booster and as a way to ease coughing and the effects of laryngitis.

This is a relatively safe and stable oil. No real precautions except not to misuse or abuse as are the case with all essential oils.

Bay Laurel Oil

This has a fruity and fresh aroma to it. Different from normal bay oil this essential oil is perfect for emotional support and promoting a higher level of confidence and courage. This essential oil is known as a nice expectorant and therefore is perfect for use in certain diffuser blends, especially those that combat illness such as flu and colds. Other reasons for using this essential oil include tonsillitis and poor appetite.

This essential oil can lead to a higher rate of issues when it is applied topically. Use extra care when applying this essential oil on your skin. Make sure it's always properly diluted. Don't use on skin that is damaged.

Bergamot Oil

This has a citrus and floral aroma to it. This oil is known for increasing one's energy and boosting one's mood. It has a great complex citrus infused aroma that is a favorite of mine. This oil is great for treating colds sores, grief, depression, halitosis, acne, stress, acne, itching, loss of appetite, and oily skin.

This kind of essential oil is highly phototoxic and therefore once applied proper precautions must be made to avoid all UVA rays. This includes direct sunlight and tanning beds on the area treated topically for a period of 24 hours.

Black Pepper Oil

This has a crisp, fresh peppercorn aroma to it. This isn't an essential oil that I use often. It's helpful for dealing with arthritis, easing sore muscles, increasing alertness, improving digestion, increasing stamina, and relieving constipation. This essential oil should be avoided at night time as it's prone to keep you up late.

This is a relatively safe and stable essential oil. No real precautions are needed except not to misuse or abuse as are the case with all types of essential oils.

Citronella Oil

This has a nice fresh, sweet, citrus aroma to it. This oil is generally used to help fight against headaches, fatigue, oily skin, and excessive perspiration. It is also a popular insect repellent and one of my favorite ways to ward off bugs in the summertime.

This is a relatively safe and stable oil. No real precautions except not to misuse or abuse as are the case with all essential oils.

Cardamom Oil

This has a rich and woody aroma to it. This is a great oil for both therapeutic and aromatic blending. This is a very popular blending oil as it goes well with many other types of essential oils. It's known as a good expectorant that is used to help relieve stress, depression, and fatigue. It's also used to help combat a loss of appetite, halitosis, and colic.

This type of essential oil should be avoided by younger children, especially around their face. Can cause breathing problems and CNS.

Catnip Oil

This has a herb and mint aroma to it. This oil is used often as an insect repellent. This oil is generally used as an anesthetic, sedative, astringent, anti-rheumatic, and anti-inflammatory.

This essential oil can cause irritation to the skin when applied topically. Be very careful when using this oil. Do not use more than is called for in a recipe.

Carrot Seed Oil

This has a warm, earthy, and woody aroma to it. This oil is used primarily in skin care regimens. It's known for helping with damaged and mature skin. This oil is not generally used in aromatics due to its unpleasant aroma. It's more geared towards helping with issues like gout, water retention, eczema, and removal of toxins.

This type of essential oil should be avoided during both breastfeeding and pregnancy.

Cassia Oil

This has a spicy cinnamon aroma to it. This essential oil is used primarily in fragrance blends. It has an aroma similar to that of cinnamon oil. It's also known for helping with relieving gas, indigestion, diarrhea, colic, rheumatism, and colds.

This kind of essential oil should be avoided by younger children and pregnant or breastfeeding women. Can cause blood clotting issues. It can also cause irritation to the skin when applied topically. Be very careful when using this oil. Do not use more than is called for in a recipe.

Cedarwood Oil

This has a woody, sharp, and sweet aroma to it. This essential oil has been popular since the ancient Egyptians. It's known for its grounding and calming properties. This oil is generally used to combat negativity, stress, arthritis, dermatitis, coughing, bronchitis, dandruff, and as an aphrodisiac. This is a popular essential oil in masculine blends.

This is a safe and stable oil. No real precautions are needed except not to misuse or abuse as are the case with all essential oils.

Cinnamon Leaf & Bark Oil

This has a rich cinnamon aroma to it. Cinnamon leaf oil is usually less well received than cinnamon bark oil but is a cheaper alternative. These oils are often used to treat low blood pressure, flatulence, stress, constipation, scabies, lice, exhaustion, regulating blood sugar levels, reducing inflammation, rheumatism, and improving insulin sensitivity.

These kinds of essential oil can cause skin irritation and mucous membrane irritation. They should be avoided by both children and women who are pregnant or breastfeeding. Be very careful when using these oils. Do not use more than is called for in a recipe.

Eucalyptus Globulus Oil

This has a fresh strong earthy aroma to it. It's great for dealing with the flu, fever, coughing, arthritis, poor circulation, colds, cold sores, and bronchitis.

This essential oil should not be used around young children, especially near their faces as it can cause breathing issues and CNS. This essential oil should not be ingested as it can be toxic when taken internally.

Clary Sage Oil

This has an earthy & bright aroma to it. I often use this in my diffuser blends. This oil is generally used to help deal with a sore throat, gas, exhaustion, stress, asthma, labor pains, and coughing.

Studies suggest one should avoid consuming alcohol when using this type of essential oil. Women with breast cancer or at higher risk for breast cancer should also steer clear of using this essential oil.

Coriander Oil

Also occasionally referred to as cilantro oil. This has a spicy, woody, and sweet aroma to it. It is used to relieve the effects of colic, arthritis, fatigue, nausea, indigestion, general aches, and rheumatism.

This is a safe and stable essential oil. No real precautions are needed except not to misuse or abuse as are the case with all essential oils.

Cumin Oil

This has an earthy and spicy aroma to it. This essential oil is normally used to relieve the effects of bad circulation, low blood pressure, fatigue, gas, indigestion, stomach cramps, colic, and relief from a toxic build up in our system.

This essential oil should be avoided by women during pregnancy.

Fennel Oil

This type of essential oil has a sweet and earthy aroma to it. It's excellent for helping to improve digestion, reduce weight gain, achieve more peaceful sleep, and suppress appetite. It's also good for healing bruises, flatulence, nausea, and halitosis.

This essential oil can inhibit blood clotting and may react poorly with medication. Women who are pregnant or breastfeeding should not use this oil.

Clove Bud Oil

This has a spicy and woody aroma. This essential oil is often used to deal with strains, sprains, arthritis, toothaches, rheumatism, and bronchitis.

This kind of essential oil can cause skin irritation and mucous membrane irritation. It can also inhibit blood clotting and should be avoided by younger children.

Fir Needle Oil

This has a woody sweet fresh aroma to it. This oil is perfect for fighting coughs, colds, flu, bronchitis, sinusitis, rheumatism, and muscle aches.

This essential oil can cause skin irritation, especially if oxidized. Be careful when applying topically.

Frankincense Oil

This has been popular since biblical times. Has a fruity and spicy aroma to it. This essential oil is great for fighting anxiety, scars, stress, coughing fits, stretch marks, and bronchitis.

This essential oil can cause skin irritation, especially if oxidized. Be careful when applying topically.

Geranium Oil

This has a fresh and sweet aroma to it. This oil is perfect for dealing with lice, acne, oily skin, menopause, and dull skin.

This essential oil can have adverse reactions when taken with some types of medication. If you're on medication always check for any drug interactions before using this oil.

German Chamomile Oil

This has a sweet and fruity aroma to it. This oil is ideal for dealing with arthritis, allergies, boils, flatulence, dermatitis, insomnia, strains, sprains, wounds, PMS, earaches, cuts, insect bites, inflamed skin, and headaches.

This essential oil may have a negative reaction when used with certain medication. If taking medication be sure to check any drug interactions before using.

Cypress Oil

This has a woody evergreen aroma to it. It's excellent to use in blends with other oils. It really helps with concentration and alertness. This oil is also used to combat hemorrhoids, oily skin, rheumatism, and excessive perspiration.

This is a relatively safe and stable oil. No real precautions except not to misuse or abuse as are the case with all essential oils.

Ginger Oil

This has a warm and spicy aroma to it. It's great for improving circulation and is a popular oil in blends for massage. This oil is ideal for fighting motion sickness and nausea. This oil is a good mood booster and is perfect for people with arthritis and muscle aches.

This essential oil is very powerful and should be used carefully. This oil has low levels of phototoxicity. Be sure to avoid sunlight and other UV rays after applying topically.

Helichrysum Oil

This has a fresh and earthy aroma to it. This is oil is ideal for boils, acne, cuts, wounds, eczema, skin irritation, dermatitis, and burns.

This is a relatively safe and stable oil. No real precautions except not to misuse or abuse as are the case with all essential oils.

Grapefruit Oil

This has a crisp, uplifting, and sweet aroma to it. This essential oil is great for curbing cravings, increasing endurance, boosting metabolism, increasing energy, reducing abdominal fat, dealing with dull skin, and reducing water retention. This essential oil also makes a nice antiseptic and disinfectant. One of my favorite essential oils.

This essential oil is highly phototoxic. Be sure to avoid sunlight and other UV rays after applying topically.

Hyssop Oil

This has a fruity, woody, and slightly sweet aroma to it. This essential oil is perfect for dealing with coughing, sore throats, and bruising. I use this one a lot whenever I'm feeling unwell.

This essential oil should be avoided by both children and by women who are pregnant or breastfeeding. Be careful when using this essential oil. Do not use more than is called for in a recipe.

Juniper Berry Oil

This oil has a sweet, crisp, and earthy aroma to it. This essential oil is ideal for dealing with gout, acne, obesity, colds, rheumatism, and lowering the number of toxins in your body. This essential oil is a natural antiseptic and can provide emotional support when diffused or burned as incense. A must have essential oil.

This is a safe and stable oil. No real precautions are needed except not to misuse or abuse as are the case with all essential oils.

Lemongrass Oil

This has an earthy and lemon aroma to it. This essential oil is used for dealing with oily skin, muscle aches, scabies, stress, acne, flatulence, excessive perspiration, and athlete's foot.

This essential oil may have negative reactions when used with certain types of medication. If taking medication be sure to check any drug interactions before using. This essential oil should be avoided by children and should not be used on skin that is damaged.

Lavender Oil

This has a sweet, fresh, and floral aroma to it. This essential oil is ideal for dealing with anxiety, sprains, allergies, strains, stress, asthma, vertigo, headaches, insect bites, earaches, burns, bruises, labor pains, oily skin, hypertension, sores, and rheumatism. This is a must own essential oil and one of the initial ones you should be adding to your inventory when starting out.

This is a safe and stable oil. No real precautions are needed except not to misuse or abuse as are the case with all essential oils.

Lemon Oil

This type of essential oil has a clean slightly sour lemon aroma to it. This oil is ideal for increasing energy levels, enhancing mood, relieving pain, suppressing weight gain, improving dull and oily skin, curing athlete's foot, and getting rid of varicose veins.

This essential oil is phototoxic when cold pressed, however, it isn't phototoxic when steam distilled. Be aware of this before exposing yourself to UV or direct sunlight.

Melissa Oil

This type of essential oil has a fresh lemon aroma to it. This oil is great for fragrances, eczema, hypertension, depression, nausea, indigestion, asthma, insomnia, bronchitis, insect repellent, migraines, and menstrual cramping.

This essential oil may have a negative reaction when used with certain medication. If taking medication be sure to check any drug interactions before using. This oil should be avoided by children and should not be used on damaged skin.

Lime Oil

This has a tart and slightly citrus aroma to it. This essential oil is affordable unlike many of the more expensive essential oils on this list. That makes it an ideal oil to add to your collection. This essential oil is mainly used for dealing with the flu, varicose veins, dull skin, acne, colds, and asthma.

This essential oil is phototoxic when cold pressed, however, it isn't phototoxic when steam distilled. Be aware of this before exposing yourself to UV or direct sunlight.

Marjoram Oil

This has a medicinal woody aroma to it. This oil is good for sprains, flatulence, excessive sex drive, muscle cramps, coughing, stress, hypertension, colic, bronchitis, ticks, and aching muscles.

This is a safe and stable oil. No real precautions are needed except not to misuse or abuse as are the case with all essential oils.

Myrtle Oil

This has a slightly floral sweet aroma to it. This essential oil is good for a sore throat, asthma, and coughs.

This essential oil may have a negative reaction when used with certain medication. If taking medication be sure to check any drug interactions before using. Research suggests this oil may be carcinogenic.

Myrrh Oil

This has a warm, woody, earthy, and warm aroma to it. This essential oil is great for oral health and is used in rinses, toothpaste, and mouthwash. This essential oil also helps deal with chapped skin, ringworm, bronchitis, toothache, itching, hemorrhoids, gum care, halitosis, and athlete's foot.

This essential oil is fetotoxic and therefore should not be used by a woman who is pregnant or breastfeeding.

Orange Oil

This has a sweet orange aroma to it. This is an affordable and popular essential oil. It is ideal for slow digestion, stress, gums, flatulence, colds, constipation, and dull skin. Orange oil is nice for brightening one's mood and is great for use in cleaning product recipes.

This is a relatively safe and stable oil. No real precautions are needed except not to misuse or abuse as are the case with all essential oils.

Neroli Oil

This has an intense floral and sweet aroma to it. This essential oil is ideal for dealing with depression, stress, stretch marks, scars, insomnia, mature skin, and shock.

This is a safe and stable oil. No real precautions are needed except not to misuse or abuse as are the case with all essential oils.

Opoponax Oil

This has a woody deep aroma to it. This essential oil is ideal as an antispasmodic and antiseptic. This essential oil is known to help balance and mellow out emotions. It's used in incense and spiritual applications.

This essential oil is phototoxic. Be sure to avoid sunlight and other UV rays after applying topically. This oil is also a skin irritant and must be used with caution.

Oregano Oil

This has a sharp and herb like aroma. This essential oil is good for both digestion and coughing.

This essential oil should be avoided by both children and by women who are pregnant or breastfeeding. This oil can cause skin irritation and mucous membrane irritation. This oil can also lead to blood clotting issues. Be very careful when using these oils. Do not use more than is called for in a recipe.

Palmarosa Oil

This has a sweet floral fresh aroma to it. This essential oil is ideal for hydrating the skin, aiding in digestion, and emotional contentment. Palmarosa oil has strong antiseptic and antibacterial properties. It's great at combating nervousness, fatigue, and stress related conditions.

This essential oil may have negative reactions when used with certain medication. If taking medication be sure to check any drug interactions before using.

Niaouli Oil

This has a harsh, musty, earthy aroma to it. This essential oil is great for treating colds, bronchitis, coughs, whooping cough, oily skin, sore throats, flu, acne, and aches.

This essential oil should not be used around young children, especially near their faces as it can cause breathing issues and CNS.

Palo Santo Oil

This has a woody sweet yet slightly minty aroma to it. This essential oil is ideal for eliciting a sense of calm and serenity. It works great at fighting depression, anxiety, emotional trauma, colds, coughs, respiratory ailments, and even as an insect repellent.

This essential oil can cause skin irritation when applied topically. Be very careful when using these oils. Do not use more than is called for in a recipe.

Peppermint Oil

This has a minty fresh aroma to it. This essential oil is known for having a cooling and calm effect. This oil is ideal for increasing mental alertness, increasing energy levels, aiding in digestion, reducing appetite, and elevating mood. This oil is also good for treating tension headaches, flatulence, scabies, vertigo, colic, and asthma. This essential oil is often considered to be an aphrodisiac.

This essential oil can cause skin irritation and mucous membrane irritation. This oil should not be used on children or people with certain medical heart conditions.

Parsley Oil

This has a woody aroma to it. This essential oil is great for indigestion, frigidity, arthritis, and rheumatism.

This essential oil should be avoided by women who are pregnant or breastfeeding. This essential oil may have negative reactions when used with certain medication. If taking medication be sure to check any drug interactions before using.

Patchouli Oil

This has a rich earthy aroma to it. This essential oil is great for skin care and is perfect in diffuser blends for romance. This is a favorite of mine. This essential oil is ideal for stress, mature skin, oily skin, eczema, dermatitis, acne, chapped skin, athlete's foot, and as an insect repellent.

This essential oil may have a negative reaction when used with certain medication. If taking medication be sure to check any drug interactions before using. This oil may also inhibit blood clotting. Always be sure to use this oil carefully.

Petitgrain Oil

This has a fresh floral aroma to it. This essential oil is ideal for people dealing with stress, acne, fatigue, and oily skin. This essential oil is great for improving mood and providing a burst of energy.

This is a safe and stable oil. No real precautions are needed except not to misuse or abuse as are the case with all essential oils.

Ravensara Oil

This has a sweet and medicinal aroma to it. This essential oil is great for dealing with cold sores, joint pain, influenza, shingles, muscle pain, colds, and bronchitis.

Only use Ravensara oil that comes from the leaf. Do not use if it comes from the bark. This oil can cause skin irritation if not used properly.

Rose Geranium Oil

This has a floral aroma to it. This essential oil is ideal for dealing with menopause, lice, dull skin, acne, and oily skin.

This essential oil may have a negative reaction when used with certain medication. If taking medication be sure to check any drug interactions before using.

Roman Chamomile Oil

This has a crisp, fruity, and bright aroma to it. This essential oil is great for the sense of calm it can bring to those using it. This essential oil is ideal for dealing with insomnia, stress, arthritis, nausea, sprains, cuts, strains, boils, flatulence, earaches, headaches, colic, sores, inflamed skin, rheumatism, insect bites, allergies, and abscesses.

This is a safe and stable oil. No real precautions are needed except not to misuse or abuse as are the case with all essential oils.

Rosewood Oil

This sweet, fruity, and woody aroma to it. Rosewood is a great aromatic oil. This essential oil is ideal for dealing with sensitive skin, flu, stress, scars, acne, fever, colds, and stretch marks.

This is a safe and stable oil. No real precautions are needed except not to misuse or abuse as are the case with all essential oils.

Rosemary Oil

This has a fresh, sweet, and medicinal aroma to it. This essential oil is perfect for our emotional well-being and can help to boost mood, stimulate the mind, and invigorate the soul. This essential oil is excellent for skin care and hair care. This oil is ideal for dealing with gout, poor circulation, exhaustion, aching muscles, dandruff, arthritis, muscles cramps, and rheumatism.

This essential oil is potentially neurotoxic and should be not be used on children. This oil can cause skin irritation if not used properly.

Spruce Oil

This has a sweet, earthy, and woody aroma to it. This essential oil is great for dealing with depression and coughing.

This is a safe and stable oil. No real precautions are needed except not to use the oil once it has gotten old and oxidized.

Sandalwood Oil

This has a rich, delicate, and sweet aroma to it. Sandalwood is perfect for instilling a sense of calm and inner peace. This essential oil is ideal for dealing with scars, oily skin, stretch marks, depression, bronchitis, laryngitis, dry skin, and stress.

This essential oil can cause skin irritation in rare instances. Be careful not to misuse or abuse the use of this essential oil.

Spearmint Oil

This has a minty and fruity aroma to it. This essential oil is great for easing tension and headaches. This oil is ideal for exhaustion, asthma, scabies, vertigo, flatulence, and fever.

This essential oil can cause skin irritation and mucous membrane irritation. Always be sure to use this oil carefully.

Vetiver Oil

This has a woody, smokey, and earthy aroma to it. This essential oil is ideal for spiritual and emotional applications. Vetiver oil is strong and should always be diluted. This essential oil is ideal for dealing with stress, cuts, rheumatism, arthritis, depression, sores, rheumatism, insomnia, oily skin, and acne.

This essential oil can cause skin irritation in some instances. Be careful not to misuse or abuse the use of this essential oil.

Tree Tea Oil

This has a medicinal and earthy aroma to it. Tree tea is one of my favorite oils. This oil is ideal for cold sores, warts, candida, insect bites, oily skin, whooping cough, colds, flu, itching, migraines, and sinusitis.

This essential oil can cause skin irritation in rare instances. Be careful not to misuse or abuse the use of this essential oil.

Thyme Oil

This has a fresh and medicinal aroma to it. This essential oil is ideal for dealing with MRSA, colds, cuts, arthritis, oily skin, lice, poor circulation, sore throat, laryngitis, muscle aches, and dermatitis.

This is a safe and stable oil. No real precautions are needed except not to misuse or abuse as are the case with all essential oils.

Ylang Ylang Oil

This has a fruity, sweet, and floral aroma to it. This essential oil is ideal for combating acne and oily skin, reducing stress, and as an aphrodisiac. This essential oil is good for dealing with hypertension, anxiety, depression, stress, and palpitations.

This essential oil should be avoided by children. This oil can cause skin irritation and should not be used on damaged skin or hypersensitive skin.

Yarrow Oil

This has a sharp woody aroma to it. This essential oil is ideal for dealing with scars, hair care, indigestion, insomnia, fever, varicose veins, hypertension, wounds, hemorrhoids, and stretch marks.

This essential oil may have a negative reaction when used with certain medication. If taking medication be sure to check any drug interactions before using. This oil is also potentially neurotoxic and can cause skin irritation in some cases.

Chapter Five: 200+ Essential Oils Recipes

Essential Oils Recipes For Your Home

In this section, I'm going to give you some recipes that are great for around your home. I use many of these on a consistent basis.

1. Insect Away! Diffuser Recipe

2 Drops of Thyme Oil

2 Drops of Lemon Grass Oil

2 Drops of Basil Oil

2 Drops of Eucalyptus Oil

Directions:

Add these oils to your diffuser and say goodbye to insects.

2. Pet Dander Diffuser Recipe

3 Drops of Peppermint Oil

2 Drops of Ginger Oil

1 Drop of Thyme Oil

Directions:

Add these oils to your diffuser. Use as needed in rooms frequented by your pets.

3. Goodbye Odor Diffuser Recipe

2 Drops of Lemon Oil

1 Drop of Melaleuca Oil

1 Drop of Lime Oil

1 Drop of Cilantro Oil

Directions:

Add these oils to your diffuser and enjoy a cleaner smelling home.

4. Insect Repellent Diffuser Recipe

1 Drop of Melaleuca Oil

1 Drop of Lemon Grass Oil

1 Drop of Rosemary Oil

1 Drop of Eucalyptus Oil

1 Drop of Thyme Oil

Directions:

Add these oils to your diffuser and say goodbye to insects.

5. All Purpose Cleaner Recipe

3 Drops of Eucalyptus Oil

2 Drops of Rosemary Oil

Directions:

Mix all your ingredients together and add to a bottle 3/4 filled with water. Spray on areas as needed.

6. Floor Cleaner Recipe

1 Quart of Water

1/4 Cup of Distilled White Vinegar

3 Drops of Eucalyptus Oil

2 Drops of Lemongrass Oil

Mix your water and white vinegar together. Add the essential oils. Apply to your floor using a mop. Rinse with clean water after applied for a few minutes.

7. Anti-Microbial Recipe

1 Tablespoon of Jojoba Oil

3 Drops of Rosemary Oil

2 Drops of Lemongrass Oil

1 Drop of Thyme Oil

Directions:

Mix all your ingredients together and apply to surfaces in your home that need cleaning.

8. Beat Stains Recipe

2 Drops of Lemongrass Oil

Directions:

Rub your oil onto your stain and allow to set for a few minutes. Place in your washing machine.

9. Laundry Recipe

25 Drops of Eucalyptus Oil

Laundry Detergent

Directions:

Add your oil to your laundry detergent and shake well to mix together. Use on clothes.

10. Litter Box Cleaner Recipe

1 Cup of White Vinegar

2 Drops of Lavender Oil

Directions:

Use vinegar while cleaning the litter box. Then dilute your lavender in a bottle of water. Rinse your litter box out with this water mixture.

11. Window Cleaner Recipe

1 Cup of White Vinegar

10 Drops of Lemon Oil

Water

Add your water and white vinegar to a spray bottle until it is 3/4 of the way full. Shake it well to combine. Add the lemon oil and shake again to combine. Spray on any windows that need cleaning and wipe off with your paper towel.

12. Bugs Away! Diffuser Recipe

1 Drop of Eucalyptus Oil

1 Drop of Thyme Oil

1 Drop of Lemongrass Oil

1 Drop of Basil Oil

Directions:

Add these oils to your diffuser and say goodbye to insects.

Essential Oil Recipes for Skincare

In this section, I'll be giving you a few recipes that are perfect for all types of skincare. Try these out whenever the situation demands. I use many of these on a normal basis and have had excellent results over the years. I hope they help to serve you just as well.

1. Whipped Coconut Oil Cellulite Cream Recipe

1 Cup of Pure Organic Coconut Oil

15 Drops of Young Living Lemon Oil

5 Drops of Young Living Peppermint Oil

Directions:

In your glass bowl, combine coconut oil with your essential oils. Mix together well using your metal whisk until your mixture has a whipped appearance.

2. Hair & Scalp Recipe

30 ML of Jojoba Oil

8 Drops of Rosemary Oil

4 Drops of Peppermint Oil

4 Drops of Cypress

4 Drops of Lavender

<u>Directions:</u>

Mix all your ingredients together and apply topically as needed.

3. Perfect Skin Body Butter Recipe

2 ounces of Shea Butter

2 ounces of Evening Primrose Oil

10 Drops of Young Living Frankincense Oil

10 Drops of Young Living Jasmine Oil

<u>Directions:</u>

In your double boiler, melt your shea butter until it is a liquid (but let it get hot!). Before you add your evening primrose oil, make sure that your shea butter isn't hot. It should be room temperature or slightly warmer. Add your evening primrose oil and blend well using a hand mixer with a whisk attachment. Place your mixture in your fridge for a few minutes until it is cool but not solidified. Remove from your fridge, use a hand mixer on high speed to whip your oils into a white colored cream. It should turn into the texture similar to that of pancake batter. Add your essential oils, and mix on a low speed with a hand mixer until they are well-combined. Pour into glass containers with lids. The mixture will set and become the texture of butter.

4. Regenerative Skin Blend Recipe

15 ML of Rose Hip Seed Oil & Tamanu Oil (50/ 50 Mix)

12 Drops of Helichrysum Italicum Oil

6 Drops of Rosemary Verbenone Oil

6 Drops of Carrot Seed Oil

Directions:

Mix all your ingredients together and apply topically as needed.

5. Homemade Stretch Mark Cream Recipe

1 Cup of Organic Unrefined Coconut Oil

1 Tablespoon of Vitamin E Oil

15 Drops of Frankincense Oil

15 Drops of Lavender Oil

Directions:

Combine all of your ingredients and beat for approximately 5 minutes using an electric mixer. Your consistency will be whipped and look like lotion. Store in a 1/2 pint mason jar.

6. Oily Skin Treatment Recipe

1 Tablespoon of Coconut Butter

6 Drops of Tea Tree Oil

6 Drops of Lavender

2 Drops of Yarrow

Directions:

Mix all your ingredients together and apply topically as needed.

7. Troubled Skin Treatment Recipe

3 Tablespoons of Rose Hip Seed Oil

1 Drop of Yarrow

1 Drop of Myrtle

1 Drop of Tea Tree

1 Drop of Lavender

Directions:

Mix all your ingredients together and apply topically as needed.

8. Dry Skin Assistance Recipe

15 ML of Argan

8 Drops of Rose Oil

4 Drops of Vetiver Oil

4 Drops of Sandalwood Oil

Directions:

Mix all your ingredients together and apply topically as needed.

9. Rough Heels & Feet Blend Recipe

15 ML of Jojoba Oil

6 Drops of German Chamomile Oil

6 Drops of Carrot Seed Oil

3 Drops of Tagetes Oil

Directions:

Mix all your ingredients together and apply before bedtime as needed.

10. Leg Circulation Recipe

1/2 Ounce of Carrier Oil

2 Drops of Chamomile

2 Drops of Geranium

2 Drops of Cypress

2 Drops of Yarrow

Directions:

Mix all your ingredients together and dot on affected areas as needed.

11. Younger Skin Assist Recipe

1 Tablespoon of Rose Hip Seed Oil

3 Drops of Tea Tree Oil

3 Drops of Lavender

2 Drops of Yarrow

2 Drops of Myrtle

Directions:

Mix all your ingredients together and apply topically as needed.

12. Better Skin Blend Recipe

1 Ounce of Jojoba

7 Drops of Cypress Oil

5 Drops of Geranium

2 Drops of Cape Chamomile

Directions:

Mix all your ingredients together and apply topically as needed.

13. Stretch Mark Help Recipe

15 ML Rose Hip Seed Oil & Tamanu Oil (50/50 Mix)

10 Drops of Helichrysum Oil

6 Drops of Clementine Oil

3 Drops of Neroli Oil

3 Drops of Lavender Oil

Directions:

Mix all your ingredients together and apply topically as needed. Avoid direct sunlight once applied.

14. Mature Skin Assist Recipe

1 Ounce of Rose Hip Seed Oil

7 Drops of Cistus Oil

4 Drops of Frankincense / Myrrh Oil Distillation

4 Drops of Helichrysum Oil

2 Drops of Chamomile

Directions:

Mix all your ingredients together and apply topically as needed.

15. Clearer Nails Blend Recipe

30 ML of Jojoba Oil

8 Drops of Tea Tree Oil

4 Drops of Myrrh Oil

4 Drops of Tagetes Oil

Directions:

Mix all your ingredients together and apply topically to any affected areas.

16. Clear Toenail Soak Recipe

6 Drops of Palmarosa Oil

3 Drops of Patchouli Oil

3 Drops of Lemongrass Oil

2 Drops of Tea Tree Oil

Directions:

Mix all your ingredients together and add to a warm foot bath.

17. Injured Skin Treatment Recipe

1 Ounce of Rose Hip Seed Oil

3 Drops of St. John's Wort

3 Drops of Helichrysum Oil

2 Drops of Roman Chamomile Oil

Directions:

Mix all your ingredients together and apply topically as needed. Avoid direct sunlight once applied.

18. Facial Toner Mist Recipe

2 Ounces of Rose Hydrosol

4 Drops of Yarrow Oil

4 Drops of Patchouli Oil

2 Drops of Cypress Oil

2 Drops Sandalwood Oil

Directions:

Mix all your ingredients together and apply as needed.

19. Facial Revitalizing Blend Recipe

15 ML of Jojoba Oil

5 Drops of Vitamin E Oil

8 Drops of Wild Carrot Seed

4 Drops of Helichrysum Italicum Oil

2 Drops of Frankincense Oil

2 Drops of Sandalwood Oil

Directions:

Mix all your ingredients together and apply topically as needed.

20. Repair Your Skin Blend Recipe

15 ML of Aloe Vera Gel

4 Drops of Helichrysum Oil

4 Drops of Lavender Oil

2 Drops of Rose Oil

Directions:

Mix all your ingredients together and apply topically as needed.

21. Combination Skin Cream Recipe

1/2 Ounce of Facial Moisturizer

3 Drops of Geranium Oil

3 Drops of Ylang Ylang Oil

Directions:

Mix all your ingredients together and apply on areas as needed.

22. Acne Away Recipe

30 ML of Borage Seed Oil

8 Drops of Lavender Oil

7 Drops of Tea Tree Oil

2 Drops of Chamomile Oil

2 Drops of Geranium Oil

2 Drops of Juniper Oil

Directions:

Mix all your ingredients together and apply sparingly on areas as needed twice each day for six weeks. If no results try increasing the concentration of the tea tree oil and lavender oil by a few drops.

23. Dermatitis Remedy Recipe

3 Drops of Frankincense Oil

2 Drops of Orange Oil

1 Drop of Tea Tree Oil

Directions:

Mix all your ingredients together and apply onto a tissue. Rub tissue over the affected areas as needed for a few minutes.

24. Bad Make-Up Reaction Recipe

1 Tablespoon of Coconut Oil

3 Drops of Rose Oil

2 Drops of Bergamot Oil

1 Drop of Orange Oil

Directions:

Mix all your ingredients together. Massage mixture onto affected areas of your face. Do not get into your eyes, nose or mouth.

25. Jaundice Remedy Recipe

1 Tablespoon of Extra Virgin Olive Oil

2 Drops of Geranium Oil

2 Drops of Rosemary Oil

1 Drop of Lemon Oil

Directions:

Mix all your ingredients together. Massage mixture onto affected areas as needed.

26. Better Nail Growth Recipe

1 Tablespoon of Coconut Oil

1 Drop of Rose Oil

1 Drop of Lavender Oil

Directions:

Mix all your ingredients together. Apply mixture to your bare nails on a daily basis

27. Skin Inflammation Recipe

1 Tablespoon of Coconut Oil

3 Drops of Frankincense Oil

2 Drops of Rosewood Oil

Directions:

Mix all your ingredients together. Dab onto a cotton ball and apply to your affected area as needed.

28. Sores Relief Recipe

1 Tablespoon of Coconut Oil

3 Drops of Lavender Oil

3 Drops of Rosewood Oil

Directions:

Mix all your ingredients together. Gently massage your mixture into your sores. Do this daily until the sores are healed.

29. Dry Skin Day Cream Recipe

80 ML of Aqueous Cream

10 ML of Rose Hip Oil

10 ML of Aloe Vera Gel

10 Drops of Palmarosa Oil

5 Drops of Sandalwood Oil

5 Drops of Geranium Oil

5 Drops of Lavender Oil

5 Drops of Jasmine Oil

Directions:

Mix all your ingredients together. Clean skin and pat dry. Apply your mixture.

30. Dry Hair Conditioner Recipe

25 ML of Jojoba Oil (Warmed up slightly)

5 Drops of Lavender Oil

5 Drops of Vetiver Oil

Directions:

Mix your ingredients together. Apply the mixture to your scalp and massage it in. Wrap your head in a cling wrap for approximately 20 minutes before rinsing mixture out.

31. Night Moisturizer Treatment Recipe

80 ML of Rose Hip Oil

5 Drops of Neroli Oil

5 Drops of Sandalwood Oil

5 Drops of Lavender Oil

5 Drops of Rose Oil

Directions:

Mix all your ingredients together. Clean face and pat dry. Apply your mixture.

32. Overnight Healing Treatment Recipe

100 ML of Rose Hip Oil

10 ML of Avocado Oil

5 Drops of Geranium Oil

5 Drops of Rose Oil

5 Drops of Sandalwood Oil

5 Drops of Lavender Oil

5 Drops of Neroli Oil

Directions:

Mix all your ingredients together. Clean face and pat dry. Place 1 dot of mixture on each cheek and dab it in. Place another 2 dots of mixture to cover your temples and forehead. Place another 3 dots on your neck. Place another dot on the back of each of your hands. Place a warm washcloth over your face. Relax for 10 minutes. Remove any mixture and dab your skin dry.

33. Cleaner Pores Steam Treatment Recipe

2 Drops of Tea Tree Oil

2 Drops of Lemon Oil

Directions:

Mix your ingredients together. Add your mixture to steaming water. Place a towel over your head and place head over the bowl. Be sure to keep eyes closed. After 5 minutes remove towel and wash off face of any debris.

34. Oily Skin Steam Treatment Recipe

2 Drops of Lavender Oil

2 Drops of Juniper Oil

Directions:

Mix your ingredients together. Add your mixture to steaming water. Place a towel over your head and place head over the bowl. Be sure to keep eyes closed. After 5 minutes remove towel and wash off face of any debris.

35. Relieve Sunburn Recipe

1 Tablespoon of Avocado Oil

1 Drop of Eucalyptus Oil

1 Drop of Peppermint Oil

Directions:

Mix all your ingredients together. Apply mixture to your affected areas until healed.

36. Oily Hair Conditioner Recipe

25ML of Olive Oil (Warmed up slightly)

5 Drops of Lavender Oil

5 Drops of Rosemary Oil

Directions:

Mix your ingredients together. Apply the mixture to your scalp and massage it in. Wrap your head in a cling wrap for approximately 20 minutes before rinsing mixture out.

37. Scalp Rub Treatment Recipe

5 Drops of Tea Tree Oil

5 Drops of Lavender Oil

Directions:

Mix your ingredients together. Apply the mixture to your scalp and massage it in.

38. Acne Mask Recipe

25 ML of Clay Paste (Water mixed with clay)

2 Drops of Rose Oil

2 Drops of Bergamot Oil

2 Drops of Tea Tree Oil

Directions:

Mix all your ingredients together. Apply mixture to your face for approximately 15 minutes before washing off.

Essential Oils Recipes for Flu, Colds, & Congestion

In this section, I'll be giving you some recipes that are perfect for treating all different types of flu, colds, and congestion. Try these out whenever you're beginning to feel under the weather. I use many of these throughout the year and they always help to bring me some needed relief. I hope they are able to do the same for you.

1. Clear Airways Recipe

1 Ounce of Carrier Oil

4 Drops of Frankincense Oil

4 Drops of Juniper Berry Oil

2 Drops of Cedar Oil

2 Drops of Eucalyptus Oil

Directions:

Mix all your ingredients together and rub on your chest as needed.

2. Flu Diffuser Blend Recipe

2 Drops of Lavender Oil

2 Drops of Eucalyptus Oil

2 Drops of Tea Tree Oil

Directions:

Add these oils to your diffuser before going to bed.

3. Increased Immune System Diffuser Recipe

2 Drops of Lemon Oil

2 Drops of Eucalyptus Oil

1 Drop of Clove Oil

1 Drop of Lime Oil

1 Drop of Rosemary Oil

Directions:

Add these oils to your diffuser and enjoy a healthier immune system.

4. Immune Spike Diffuser Recipe

1 Drop of Wild Orange Oil

1 Drop of Cinnamon Bark Oil

1 Drop of Eucalyptus Oil

1 Drop of Clove Oil

1 Drop of Rosemary Oil

Directions:

Add these oils to your diffuser and enjoy a healthier immune system.

5. Respiratory Wellness Diffuser Recipe

2 Drops of Peppermint Oil

1 Drop of Eucalyptus Oil

1 Drop of Lemon Oil

1 Drop of Rosemary Oil

Directions:

Add these oils to your diffuser and enjoy better respiratory wellness.

6. Congested Chest Relief Recipe

1 Tablespoon of Extra Virgin Olive Oil

2 Drops of Niaouli Oil

1 Drop of Lavender Oil

1 Drop of Sweet Birch Oil

Directions:

Mix all your ingredients together and store in a dark colored bottle. Massage mixture onto your chest before bed as needed.

7. Earache Relief Recipe

1 Tablespoon of Jojoba Oil

2 Drops of Roman Chamomile Oil

2 Drops of Sandalwood Oil

Directions:

Mix all your ingredients together. Place 2 to 3 drops in the affected ear 3 times a day as needed.

8. Persistent Cough Remedy Recipe

3 Tablespoons of Honey

2 Drops of Lemon Oil

1 Drop of Eucalyptus Oil

1 Drop of Peppermint Oil

Directions:

Mix all your ingredients together. Take them orally every three hours as needed.

9. Relieve Nasal Congestion Recipe

3 Drops of Sweet Orange Oil

2 Drops of Lemon Oil

1 Blank Inhaler

Directions:

Mix all your ingredients together. Add to your inhaler and inhale deeply several times as needed.

10. Flu Reliever Recipe

1 Tablespoon of Grape Seed Oil

2 Drops of Geranium Oil

1 Drop of Sandalwood Oil

1 Drop of Lemon Oil

Directions:

Mix all your ingredients together and shake well. Apply mixture to the sides of the nose and underneath your jawline.

11. Ear Infection Remedy Recipe

1 Tablespoon of Coconut Oil

2 Drops of Peppermint Oil

1 Drop of Rose Oil

1 Drop of Lavender Oil

Directions:

Mix all your ingredients together. Rub your mixture on the outside of your ears and down your neck to help treat any infection.

12. Influenza Relief Recipe

500 ML of Boiling Water

2 Drops of Eucalyptus Oil

1 Drop of Sandalwood Oil

1 Drop of Lavender Oil

1 Drop of Lemon Oil

Directions:

Add all your ingredients to the boiling water. Pour into a steam basin. Place your head over the basin and cover using a towel. Inhale deeply. Do this twice a day until symptoms are gone.

13. Infection Begone Recipe

250 ML of Epsom Salts

125 ML of Baking Soda

125 ML of Milk

2 Drops of Sweet Orange Oil

2 Drops of Juniper Berry Oil

2 Drops of Eucalyptus Oil

Directions:

Draw a hot bath. Run your baking soda and Epsom salt under the bath water so it gets dissolved. Mix your essential oils and milk together. Add your mixture to the bath. Soak for approximately 30 minutes.

14. Pink Eye Remedy Recipe

1 Teaspoon of Coconut Oil

2 Drops of Lavender Oil

2 Drops of Tea Tree Oil

Directions:

Mix all your ingredients together. Apply around your eyes. Do not get in eyes. If any of the mixture gets into your eyes do not rinse them with water. Instead, rinse them with olive oil or coconut oil.

15. Flu Beater Treatment Recipe

80 ML of Sweet Almond Oil

3 Drops of Mandarin Oil

3 Drops of Tea Tree Oil

3 Drops of Eucalyptus Oil

Directions:

Mix all your ingredients together. Massage mixture into your feet, chest, and back. Use this immediately before bedtime.

16. Fever Remover Recipe

1 Drop of Eucalyptus Oil

1 Drop of Tea Tree Oil

1 Drop of Peppermint Oil

Directions:

Draw a lukewarm bath. Add your oils to the bath. Soak in the mixture until feeling less feverish or you feel cold chills.

17. Immune Booster Diffuser Recipe

2 Drops of Wild Orange Oil

2 Drops of Cinnamon Oil

2 Drops of Eucalyptus Oil

2 Drops of Clove Oil

2 Drops of Rosemary Oil

Directions:

Add these oils to your diffuser and enjoy a healthier immune system.

18. Fever Foot Rub Recipe

60 ML of Sweet Almond Oil

2 Drops of Tea Tree Oil

2 Drops of Lemon Oil

2 Drops of Eucalyptus Oil

Directions:

Mix all your ingredients together. Gently massage the mixture into the soles of each foot. Rub a small amount of the mixture onto your back and chest. Apply 3 times a day as needed.

19. Seasonal Support Inhaler Recipe

5 Drops of Lavender Oil

5 Drops of Lemon Oil

5 Drops of Peppermint Oil

Directions:

Remove wick and add the essential oils blend. To use remove the cover. Place inhaler close to your nose and inhale deeply. Use when needed.

20. Immune Booster Inhaler Recipe

3 Drops of Tea Tree Oil

3 Drops of Oregano Oil

3 Drops of Lemon Oil

3 Drops of Cinnamon Oil

3 Drops of Frankincense Oil

Directions:

Remove wick and add the essential oils blend. To use remove the cover. Place inhaler close to your nose and inhale deeply. Use when needed.

21. Deep Breath Inhaler Recipe

4 Drops eucalyptus essential oil

4 Drops peppermint essential oil

2 Drops lemon essential oil

2 Drops of Lavender Oil

2 Drops of Rosemary Oil

Directions:

Remove wick and add the essential oils blend. To use remove the cover. Place inhaler close to your nose and inhale deeply. Use when needed.

Essential Oils Recipes for Pains, Aches, & Common Ailments

In this section, I'll be giving you some recipes that will help to ease all different types of pains, aches, and common ailments. The older I become the more I find a use for these recipes. Try these out whenever you feel the need. Hopefully, you'll find these recipes as helpful as I have over the last few years.

1. Arthritis Ease Recipe

1 Tablespoon of Macadamia Nut Oil

2 Drops of Roman Chamomile Oil

1 Drop of Peppermint Oil

1 Drop of Eucalyptus Oil

1 Drop of Lavender Oil

Directions:

Mix all your ingredients together and massage on areas of your body as needed.

2. Anti-Bacterial Relief Recipe

3 Drops of Citronella Oil

2 Drops of Tea Tree Oil

1 Drop of Coconut Oil

1 Drop of Rosemary Oil

1 Drop of Lavender Oil

Directions:

Mix all your ingredients together and apply on areas of your body as needed.

3. Allergy Relief Recipe

3 Drops of Eucalyptus Oil

2 Drops of Sandalwood Oil

2 Drops of Rosemary Oil

1 Blank Inhaler

Directions:

Add all your ingredients to your blank inhaler and use inhaler whenever struck with allergy or hay fever attack.

4. Asthma Relief Recipe

15 ML of Macadamia Nut Oil

6 Drops of Lavender Oil

3 Drops of Eucalyptus Oil

3 Drops of Rosemary Oil

1 Drop of Ginger Oil

Directions:

Mix all your ingredients together in a dark glass bottle. Shake well. Massage mixture onto your back and chest on a daily basis.

5. Improved Blood Circulation Recipe

1 Tablespoon of Primrose Oil

3 Drops of Marjoram Oil

2 Drops of Goldenrod Oil

1 Drop of Cypress Oil

Directions:

Mix all your ingredients together and apply on different parts of your body. I recommend the wrists, upper back, calves, and chest areas.

6. Heal Chapped Lips Recipe

1 Tablespoon of Coconut Oil

1 Drop of Rosewood Oil

1 Drop of Roman Chamomile Oil

Directions:

Mix all your ingredients together and apply on lips as many times as needed each day until your chapped lips are gone.

7. Dust Allergy Diffuser Recipe

3 Drops of Melissa Oil

1 Drop of Basil Oil

1 Drop of Geranium Oil

Directions:

Mix all your ingredients together. Add this mixture to your diffuser in the room you spend the most time in.

8. Detoxify Yourself Diffuser Recipe

1 Tablespoon of Macadamia Nut Oil

3 Drops of Juniper Oil

Directions:

Mix all your ingredients together. Add this mixture to your diffuser in the room you spend the most time in.

9. Heat Rash Relief Recipe

1 Tablespoon of Borage Oil

3 Drops of Patchouli Oil

3 Drops of Neroli Oil

Directions:

Mix all your ingredients together. Massage mixture onto your rash as needed.

10. Constipation Relief Recipe

1 Tablespoon of Coconut Oil

1 Drop of Rosemary Oil

1 Drop of Orange Oil

1 Drop of Ginger Oil

Directions:

Mix all your ingredients together and store in a dark colored bottle. Massage mixture into your stomach in a clockwise direction.

11. Hay Fever Recipe

3 Drops of Frankincense Oil

3 Drops of Peppermint Oil

1 Blank Inhaler

Directions:

Mix all your essential oils together and add to your inhaler. Inhale deeply whenever you feel an attack coming on.

12. Croup Remedy Recipe

1 Tablespoon of Avocado Oil

2 Drops of Sandalwood Oil

2 Drops of Ravensara Oil

2 Drops of Marjoram Oil

1 Drop of Thyme Oil

Directions:

Mix all your ingredients together and massage onto your chest as needed.

13. Indigestion Relief Recipe

1 Tablespoon of Coconut Oil

3 Drops of Grapeseed Oil

3 Drops of Lemongrass Oil

Directions:

Mix all your ingredients together and place them in a bottle. Inhale deeply as needed.

14. Heartache Relief

1 Tablespoon of Primrose Oil

3 Drops of Lavender Oil

2 Drops of Bergamot Oil

1 Drop of Tea Tree Oil

Directions:

Mix all your ingredients together. Massage mixture onto your chest as needed.

15. Ingrown Hair Recipe

3 Drops of Tea Tree Oil

3 Drops of Peppermint Oil

Plain Body Wash or Lotion

Directions:

Mix all your ingredients together. Shake the mixture and apply to your body as needed.

16. Intestinal Issues Recipe

5 ML of Vegetable Carrier Oil

2 Drops of Rosemary Oil

1 Drop of Clove Oil

1 Drop of Chamomile Oil

1 Drop of Peppermint Oil

Directions:

Mix all your ingredients together. Apply mixture over your stomach as needed.

17. Jaw Pain Relief

2 Tablespoons of Avocado Oil

3 Drops of Olbas Oil

1 Drop of Juniper Oil

Directions:

Mix all your ingredients together. Massage mixture into your jawline to loosen your jaw and relieve pain.

18. Overcome Nausea Recipe

3 Drops of Tarragon Oil

1 Blank Inhaler

Directions:

Add oil to your inhaler. Inhale deeply as needed.

19. Neck Strain Relief Recipe

1 Tablespoon of Avocado Oil

3 Drops of Lavender Oil

1 Drop of Rosemary Oil

Directions:

Mix all your ingredients together. Massage mixture into your strained neck area as needed.

20. Renal Function Remedy Recipe

1 Tablespoon of Coconut Oil

2 Drops of Ledum Oil

1 Drop of Celery Seed Oil

1 Drop of Carrot Seed Oil

Directions:

Mix all your ingredients together. Massage mixture gently into your sides where kidneys are located.

21. Aching Knees Recipe

1 Tablespoon of Avocado Oil

3 Drops of Ginger Oil

3 Drops of Sweet Orange Oil

Directions:

Mix all your ingredients together. Massage mixture into your knee as needed.

22. Aching Legs Recipe

1 Tablespoon of Coconut Oil

3 Drops of Marjoram Oil

2 Drops of Jasmine Oil

Directions:

Mix all your ingredients together. Massage mixture into your legs as needed.

23. Shoulder Pain Relief Recipe

1 Tablespoon of Avocado Oil

3 Drops of Sandalwood Oil

1 Drop of German Chamomile Oil

Directions:

Mix all your ingredients together. Massage mixture gently into your shoulder area several times each day.

24. Relieve Thrush Recipe

1 Tablespoon of Vegetable Oil

2 Drops of Rosewood Oil

1 Drop of Thyme Oil

1 Drop of Chamomile Oil

Directions:

Mix all your ingredients together. Apply mixture to the roof of your mouth.

25. Yeast Infection Recipe

3 Drops of Oregano Oil

2 Drops of Lavender Oil

Directions:

Mix all your ingredients together. Ingest the mixture twice a day until for up to 2 weeks until your infection is gone.

26. Swollen Ankles Relief Recipe

1 Tablespoon of Avocado Oil

3 Drops of Ginger Oil

3 Drops of Peppermint Oil

Directions:

Mix all your ingredients together. Massage mixture into your ankles as needed.

27. Improve Immunity Diffuser Blend Recipe

2 Drops of Lavender Oil

2 Drops of Tea Tree Oil

Directions:

Add oils to your diffuser and enjoy.

28. Immunity Booster Cream Recipe

50 ML of Aqueous Cream

2 Drops of Chamomile Oil

2 Drops of Lavender Oil

2 Drops of Marjoram Oil

Directions:

Mix all your ingredients together. Massage mixture into the soles of your feet each night for 2 weeks.

29. Tonsillitis Relief Recipe

1 Tablespoon of Coconut Oil

2 Drops of Ginger Oil

2 Drops of Tea Tree Oil

1 Drop of Lemon Oil

1 Drop of Lavender Oil

1 Drop of Roman Chamomile Oil

Directions:

Mix all your ingredients together. Apply mixture to the outside area of your throat and gently massage.

30. Immunity Tonic Mix Recipe

100 ML of Sweet Almond Oil

6 Drops of Bergamot Oil

6 Drops of Lavender Oil

3 Drops of Tea Tree Oil

3 Drops of Lemon Oil

2 Drops of Myrrh Oil

Directions:

Mix all your ingredients together. Massage mixture over areas of body that are prone to developing physical issues.

31. Pain Reliever Recipe

10 ML of Sweet Almond Oil

10 Ml of Jojoba Oil

2 Drops of Chamomile Oil

2 Drops of Sweet Marjoram Oil

2 Drops of Melissa Oil

Directions:

Mix all your ingredients together. Massage mixture into affected areas twice daily as needed.

32. Diaper Rash Treatment Recipe

250 ML Aqueous Cream

10 Drops of Lavender Oil

5 Drops of Palmarosa Oil

5 Drops of Geranium Oil

5 Drops of Sandalwood Oil

Directions:

Mix all your ingredients together. Apply mixture onto affected areas as needed.

33. Psoriasis Treatment Cream Recipe

200 ML of Thick Aqueous Cream

10 ML of Borage Oil

10 ML Avocado Oil

5 Drops of Tea Tree Oil

5 Drops of Myrrh Oil

5 Drops of Lavender Oil

Directions:

Mix all your ingredients together. Apply mixture onto affected areas as needed.

34. Motion Ease Inhaler Recipe

5 Drops of Peppermint Oil

4 Drops of Ginger Oil

3 Drops of Coriander Oil

3 Drops of Fennel Oil

Directions:

Remove wick and add the essential oils blend. To use remove the cover. Place inhaler close to your nose and inhale deeply. Use when needed.

Essential Oils Calming & Relaxing Recipes

In this section, I'll be giving you some recipes that will allow you to reach a state of calm and relaxation. I love to use these whenever I've had a tough or stressful day. If you need to find some inner calm and peace of mind these recipes will help do the trick.

1. Sound Asleep Diffuser Recipe

4 Drops of Cedarwood Oil

3 Drops of Lavender Oil

Directions:

Add these oils to your diffuser and sleep better.

2. Fast Asleep Diffuser Recipe

3 Drops of Balance Oil

2 Drops of Vetiver Oil

2 Drops of Roman Chamomile Oil

2 Drops of Lavender Oil

Directions:

Add these oils to your diffuser and sleep better.

3. Lights Out Diffuser Recipe

3 Drops of Lavender Oil

3 Drops of Vetiver Oil

2 Drops of Frankincense Oil

Directions:

Add these oils to your diffuser and sleep better.

4. Nighty Nite Diffuser Recipe

2 Drops of Vetiver Oil

2 Drops of Chamomile Oil

2 Drops of Lavender Oil

Directions:

Add these oils to your diffuser and sleep better.

5. Sleeping Easy Diffuser Recipe

3 Drops of Lavender Oil

2 Drops of Marjoram Oil

1 Drop of Roman Chamomile Oil

1 Drop of Orange Oil

Directions:

Add these oils to your diffuser and sleep better.

6. Chill Out Diffuser Recipe

2 Drops of Cedarwood Oil

2 Drops of Vetiver Oil

Directions:

Add these oils to your diffuser and relax.

7. Sayonara Stress Diffuser Recipe

2 Drops of Bergamot Oil

2 Drops of Frankincense Oil

Directions:

Add these oils to your diffuser and say goodbye to stress.

8. Relaxation Massage Oil Recipe

6 Teaspoons of Massage Oil Base

4 Drops of Lavender Oil

1 Drop of Frankincense Oil

1 Drop of Petitgrain Oil

Directions:

Add all your drops to 6 teaspoons of your massage oil base. Mix together. Add to your warm bath.

9. Tension Tamer Inhaler Recipe

6 Drops of Peppermint Oil

3 Drops of Frankincense Oil

3 Drops of Chamomile Oil

3 Drops of Lavender Oil

Directions:

Remove wick and add the essential oils blend. To use remove the cover. Place inhaler close to your nose and inhale deeply. Use when needed.

Essential Oils Recipes For Pleasant Smelling Blends

Diffusing your essential oils will not only make your home smell nicer, it can also provide other health benefits. I always prefer to use cold-air diffusers. I prefer them because anything that heats your oils can do damage to some of their more beneficial properties. I suggest never using candle warmers or other items that can heat the essential oils excessively. Sticking with a cold air diffuser is the best way to ensure you benefit from all the positive effects of your essential oils.

In this section, I'll be giving you some recipes that are pleasant to smell. I've tried all of these at one point or another and have greatly enjoyed them. Hopefully, you'll find a few that you enjoy as well.

Be aware the blends in this section are meant to be used in your cold-air diffuser. These types of diffusers will normally require a tiny amount of water to be added, along with any oils. Check your diffuser's directions to find out exact amounts necessary.

1. Man Cave Blend Diffuser Recipe

2 Drops of Wintergreen Oil

2 Drops of Cypress Oil

2 Drops of White Fir Oil

Directions:

Add these oils to your diffuser and enjoy.

2. Spring Seasonal Blend Diffuser Recipe

3 Drops of Roman Chamomile Oil

3 Drops of Lavender Oil

2 Drops of Geranium Oil

Directions:

Add these oils to your diffuser and enjoy.

3. Fresh Fallen Snow Diffuser Recipe

6 Drops of Grapefruit Oil

2 Drops of Pine Needle Oil

1 Drop of Wintergreen Oil

Directions:

Add these oils to your diffuser and enjoy.

4. Holiday Eggnog Diffuser Recipe

10 Drops of Vanilla Oil

2 Drops of Nutmeg Oil

1 Drop of Cinnamon Cassia Oil

Directions:

Add these oils to your diffuser and enjoy.

5. Gingerbread Man Diffuser Recipe

3 Drops of Cinnamon Cassia Oil

2 Drops of Vanilla Oil

2 Drops of Ginger Oil

1 Drop of Clove Oil

1 Drop of Nutmeg Oil

Directions:

Add these oils to your diffuser and enjoy.

6. Jolly Holly Holidays Diffuser Recipe

4 Drops of Lemon Oil

2 Drops of Cinnamon Cassia Oil

2 Drops of Ginger Oil

2 Drops of Nutmeg Oil

1 Drop of Clove Oil

Directions:

Add these oils to your diffuser and enjoy.

7. Hearts & Mistletoe Diffuser Recipe

3 Drops of Pine Needle Oil

2 Drops of Atlas Cedar Oil

2 Drops of Rosemary Oil

1 Drop of Ylang Ylang Oil

1 Drop of Juniper Berry Oil

1 Drop of Eucalyptus Globulus Oil

Directions:

Add these oils to your diffuser and enjoy.

8. It's Christmas Again Diffuser Recipe

30 Drops of Pine Needle Oil

8 Drops of Atlas Cedar Oil

3 Drops of Cypress Oil

1 Drop of Orange Oil

Directions:

Add these oils to your diffuser and enjoy.

9. Santa's Sugar Cookies Diffuser Recipe

24 Drops of Vanilla Oil

2 Drops of Tangerine Oil

2 Drops of Cinnamon Bark Oil

1 Drop of Ginger Oil

Directions:

Add these oils to your diffuser and enjoy.

10. Under The Mistletoe Diffuser Recipe

5 Drops of Balsam Fir Needle Oil

2 Drops of Atlas Cedar Oil

1 Drop of Juniper Berry Oil

Directions:

Add these oils to your diffuser and enjoy.

11. The Orchard Diffuser Recipe

12 Drops of Orange Oil

6 Drops of Patchouli Oil

4 Drops of Ginger Oil

Directions:

Add these oils to your diffuser and enjoy.

12. Welcoming Blend Diffuser Recipe

3 Drops of Rosemary Oil

3 Drops of Lemon Oil

3 Drops of Lavender Oil

Directions:

Add these oils to your diffuser and enjoy.

13. Winter Icicles Diffuser Recipes

3 Drops of Peppermint Oil

3 Drops of Pennyroyal Oil

2 Drops of Rosemary Oil

1 Drop of Tea Tree Oil

1 Drop of Eucalyptus Globulus Oil

Directions:

Add these oils to your diffuser and enjoy.

14. Fresh Air Blend Diffuser Recipe

3 Drops of Lime Oil

3 Drops of Lemon Oil

3 Drops of Melaleuca Oil

Directions:

Add these oils to your diffuser and enjoy.

15. Bliss Blend Diffuser Recipe

3 Drops of Grapefruit Oil

3 Drops of Wild Orange Oil

2 Drops of Bergamot Oil

2 Drops of Lemon Oil

Directions:

Add these oils to your diffuser and enjoy.

16. Clean Air Blend Diffuser Recipe

4 Drops of Vetiver Oil

3 Drops of Peppermint Oil

3 Drops of Lemon Oil

Directions:

Add these oils to your diffuser and enjoy.

17. Nice Air Diffuser Recipe

3 Drops of Lemon Oil

2 Drops of Cilantro Oil

2 Drops of White Fir Oil

2 Drops of Lime Oil

2 Drops of Melaleuca Oil

Directions:

Add these oils to your diffuser and enjoy.

18. Fresher Feel Diffuser Recipe

3 Drops of Lemon Oil

2 Drops of Lime Oil

2 Drops of Cilantro Oil

2 Drops of Melaleuca Oil

Directions:

Add these oils to your diffuser and enjoy.

19. Manly Musk Diffuser Recipe

3 Drops of Arborvitae Oil

3 Drops of Cypress Oil

3 Drops of Bergamot Oil

Directions:

Add these oils to your diffuser and enjoy.

20. The Candy Shop Diffuser Recipe

4 Drops of Wintergreen Oil

4 Drops of Wild Orange Oil

Directions:

Add these oils to your diffuser and enjoy.

21. Spring & Summer Diffuser Recipe

2 Drops of Peppermint Oil

2 Drops of Lemon Oil

2 Drops of Lavender Oil

Directions:

Add these oils to your diffuser and enjoy.

22. Chai Spice Diffuser Recipe

3 Drops of Cardamom Oil

2 Drops of Clove Oil

2 Drops of Cassia Oil

1 Drop of Ginger Oil

Directions:

Add these oils to your diffuser and enjoy.

23. Garden Flower Diffuser Recipe

2 Drops of Roman Chamomile Oil

2 Drops of Lavender Oil

1 Drop of Geranium Oil

Directions:

Add these oils to your diffuser and enjoy.

24. Spicy Night Diffuser Recipe

4 Drops of Wild Orange Oil

3 Drops of Cinnamon Oil

2 Drops of Clove Oil

Directions:

Add these oils to your diffuser and enjoy.

25. Christmas Magic Diffuser Recipe

4 Drops of Cinnamon Oil

4 Drops of Patchouli Oil

3 Drops of Orange Oil

2 Drops of Clove Oil

1 Drop of Ylang Ylang Oil

Directions:

Add these oils to your diffuser and enjoy.

26. Rugged Man Diffuser Recipe

2 Drops of Wintergreen Oil

2 Drops of Cypress Oil

2 Drops of White Fir Oil

Directions:

Add these oils to your diffuser and enjoy.

27. Citrus & Spice Diffuser Recipe

3 Drops of Wild Orange Oil

2 Drops of Cinnamon Bark Oil

1 Drop of Clove Oil

Directions:

Add these oils to your diffuser and enjoy.

28. Fall Bouquet Diffuser Recipe

12 Drops of Orange Oil

3 Drops of Clove Oil

3 Drops of Cinnamon Cassia Oil

2 Drops of Nutmeg Oil

Directions:

Add these oils to your diffuser and enjoy.

29. Out In The Woods Diffuser Recipe

3 Drops of Frankincense Oil

2 Drops of White Fir Oil

1 Drop of Cedarwood Oil

Directions:

Add these oils to your diffuser and enjoy.

30. Happy Holidays Diffuser Recipe

2 Drops of Wild Orange Oil

2 Drops of White Fir Oil

1 Drop of Wintergreen Oil

Directions:

Add these oils to your diffuser and enjoy.

31. Seasonal Fall Blend Diffuser Recipe

4 Drops of Wild Orange Oil

3 Drops of Cinnamon Oil

3 Drops of Ginger Oil

Directions:

Add these oils to your diffuser and enjoy.

32. Candy Cane Diffuser Recipe

3 Drops of Peppermint Oil

2 Drops of Vanilla Oil

Directions:

Add these oils to your diffuser and enjoy.

33. Candy Dream Diffuser Recipe.

2 Drops of Wintergreen Oil

2 Drops of Wild Orange Oil

Directions:

Add these oils to your diffuser and enjoy.

34. Spice & Cinnamon Diffuser Recipe

5 Drops of Vanilla Oil

1 Drop of Orange Oil

1 Drop of Nutmeg Oil

1 Drop of Clove Oil

1 Drop of Cinnamon Bark Oil

Directions:

Add these oils to your diffuser and enjoy.

35. Cinnamon Spice Diffuser Recipe

24 Drops of Cinnamon Cassia Oil

10 Drops of Ginger Oil

5 Drops of Orange Oil

4 Drops of Nutmeg Oil

Directions:

Add these oils to your diffuser and enjoy.

36. Seasonal Summertime Blend Diffuser Recipe

3 Drops of Lavender Oil

3 Drops of Grapefruit Oil

2 Drops of Spearmint Oil

2 Drops of Lemon Oil

Directions:

Add these oils to your diffuser and enjoy.

37. Autumn Breeze Diffuser Recipe

The feeling of fall weather.

8 Drops of Orange Oil

6 Drops of Sage Oil

6 Drops of Lime Oil

Directions:

Add these oils to your diffuser and enjoy.

Essential Oils Uplifting Recipes

In this section, I'm going to give you few recipes that are perfect when you need to raise your spirits or need a boost to get going.

1. Fulfill & Uplift Diffuser Recipe

10 Drops of Bergamot Oil

3 Drops of Lemon Oil

1 Drop of Lime Oil

Directions:

Add these oils to your diffuser and enjoy.

2. Burst Of Energy Diffuser Recipe

3 Drops of Rosemary

3 Drops of Peppermint

2 Drops of Grapefruit

Directions:

Add these oils to your diffuser and enjoy.

3. Energy Blend Diffuser Recipe

3 Drops of Lemon

3 Drops of Peppermint

3 Drops of Rosemary

Directions:

Add these oils to your diffuser and enjoy.

4. Wake Up Alert Diffuser Recipe

4 Drops of Peppermint

4 Drops Wild Orange

Directions:

Add these oils to your diffuser and enjoy.

5. Energy Blaster Diffuser Recipe

3 Drops of Frankincense

3 Drops of Wild Orange

2 Drops of Cinnamon

Directions:

Add these oils to your diffuser and enjoy.

6. Pure Happiness Diffuser Recipe

2 Drops of Lime

2 Drops of Peppermint

2 Drops of Frankincense

2 Drops of Wild Orange

Directions:

Add these oils to your diffuser and enjoy.

7. Happy Happy Blend Diffuser Recipe

3 Drops of Lavender

3 Drops of Bergamot

2 Drops of Geranium

Directions:

Add these oils to your diffuser and enjoy.

8. Get Energized Diffuser Recipe

2 Drops of Cinnamon Oil

2 Drops of Frankincense Oil

2 Drops of Wild Orange Oil

Directions:

Add these oils to your diffuser and enjoy.

9. Energy Shot Recipe

1 Tablespoon of Jojoba Oil

2 Drops of Roman Chamomile Oil

2 Drops of Sandalwood Oil

Directions:

Mix all your ingredients together. Massage mixture into your chest when you need a boost of energy.

10. Fatigue Relief Recipe

1 Tablespoon of Extra Virgin Olive Oil

3 Drops of Ginger Oil

3 Drops of Peppermint Oil

Directions:

Mix all your ingredients together. Massage mixture into areas of your body that are feeling fatigued.

11. Happy Place Inhaler Recipe

7 Drops of Orange Oil

4 Drops of Ylang Ylang Oil

4 Drops of Lavender Oil

Directions:

Remove wick and add the essential oils blend. To use remove the cover. Place inhaler close to your nose and inhale deeply. Use when needed.

12. Good Times Inhaler Recipe

4 Drops of White Fir Oil

3 Drops of Orange Oil

3 Drops of Grapefruit Oil

2 Drops of Tangerine Oil

2 Drops of Lemon Oil

1 Drop of Bergamot Oil

Directions:

Remove wick and add the essential oils blend. To use remove the cover. Place inhaler close to your nose and inhale deeply. Use when needed.

13. Gratitude Inhaler Recipe

5 Drops of Bergamot Oil

4 Drops of Orange Oil

3 Drops of Geranium Oil

3 Drops of White Fir Oil

Directions:

Remove wick and add the essential oils blend. To use remove the cover. Place inhaler close to your nose and inhale deeply. Use when needed.

Essential Oils Aromatic Recipes To Help With Weight Loss

Blending your essential oils together is a wonderful way to experiment using your favorite scents. It allows you to achieve the healing qualities of each of the oils while also creating new helpful blends. The blends in this section will help with dissolving fat and suppressing appetite. These are all easy to make and I suggest trying them out for yourselves to see which ones are right for you. My personal favorites are the Rejuvenating Bath and Craving Curbing Salve, while my wife enjoys the Anti-Cellulite Rub and Fat Reducing Massage.

1. Weight Loss Mint Blend Diffuser Recipe

1 Teaspoon of Coarse Sea Salt

20 Drops of Peppermint Oil

10 Drops of Bergamot Oil

4 Drops of Spearmint Oil

1 Drop of Ylang Ylang Oil

Directions:

Add everything to a small bottle or inhaler and take 3 deep, slow, long breaths. Take a quick break and repeat. Do this three time in total. Sniff hard and long in each nostril. Do this before eating or when your appetite is triggered.

2. Weight Loss Citrus Blend Recipe

1 Teaspoon of Coarse Sea Salt

30 Drops of Grapefruit Oil

4 Drops of Lemon Oil

1 Drop of Ylang Ylang Oil

Directions:

Add everything to a small bottle or inhaler and take 3 deep, slow, long breaths. Take a quick break and repeat. Do this three time in total. Sniff hard and long in each nostril. Do this before eating or when your appetite is triggered.

3. Cellulite Help Recipe

15 ML of Grape Seed Oil

6 Drops of Grapefruit Oil

4 Drops of Lemon Oil

2 Drops of Rosemary Oil

2 Drops of Cypress Oil

Directions:

Mix all your ingredients together and apply topically as needed. Avoid direct sunlight once applied.

4. Weight Loss Herbal Blend Diffuser Recipe

1 Teaspoon of Coarse Sea Salt

15 Drops of Marjoram Oil

15 Drops of Basil Oil

1 Drop of Thyme Oil

1 Drop of Oregano Oil

Directions:

Add everything to a small bottle or inhaler and take 3 deep, slow, long breaths. Take a quick break and repeat. Do this three time in total. Sniff hard and long in each nostril. Do this before eating or when your appetite is triggered.

5. Cellulite Relief Recipe

1/2 Ounce of Carrier Oil

2 Drops of Chamomile

2 Drops of Cypress Oil

2 Drops of Yarrow Oil

2 Drops of Geranium Oil

Directions:

Mix all your ingredients together and dot on areas as needed.

6. Crave Reducer Diffuser Recipe

6 Drops of Eucalyptus Oil

Directions:

Add oil to your diffuser to help cut down on cravings. Should use in the rooms where you spend the most amount of your time.

7. Cellulite Salt Scrub Recipe

1 Cup of Seal Salt

1/2 Cup of Jojoba Oil

7 Drops of Grapefruit Oil

5 Drops of Cypress Oil

3 Drops of Patchouli Oil

Directions:

Mix all your ingredients together and apply topically as needed. Avoid direct sunlight once applied.

8. Metabolism Increaser Recipe

1 Drop of Ginger Oil

1 Drop of Grapefruit Oil

1 Drop of Peppermint Oil

1 Drop of Lemon Oil

Directions:

Mix all your ingredients together. Add mixture to your first and final drink of each day.

9. Reduce Sugar Cravings

2 Drops of Roman Chamomile Oil

1 Glass of Water

Directions:.

Add oil to a glass of water before drinking. Do this several times a day.

10. Stop Over Eating Recipe

2 Drops of Grapefruit Oil

1 Glass of Water

Directions:.

Add your oil to your glass of water before eating. Do this before each meal.

11. Tummy Tamer Inhaler Recipe

4 Drops of Peppermint Oil

4 Drops of Ginger Oil

3 Drops of Fennel Oil

2 Drops of Lemon Oil

2 Drops of Coriander Oil

Directions:

Remove wick and add the essential oils blend. To use remove the cover. Place inhaler close to your nose and inhale deeply. Use when needed.

Essential Oils Emotional Support, Mind, & Balance Recipes

In this section, I'm going to give you some recipes that are ideal when you need to clear your mind and find more clarity or balance in your life.

1. Mind Soothing Diffuser Recipe

7 Drops of Frankincense Oil

6 Drops of Cistus Oil

3 Drops of Sandalwood Oil

Directions:

Add these oils to your diffuser and enjoy.

2. Palo Santo Purify Bath Recipe

1 Cup of Epsom Salt

2 Drops of Grapefruit Oil

2 Drops of Palo Santo Oil

2 Drop of Palmarosa Oil

2 Drops of Cypress Oil

Directions:

Mix all your ingredients together and add to your bath.

3. A Meditative Blend Recipe

30 ML of Jojoba Oil

8 Drops of Frankincense Myrrh Oil

6 Drops of Sandalwood Oil

3 Drops of Cedar Oil

3 Drops of Opoponax Oil

Directions:

Mix all your ingredients together and apply as needed.

4. Life Transitioning Recipe

15 ML of Marula Oil

4 Drops of Clary Sage Oil

4 Drops of Fennel Oil

2 Drops of Geranium Oil

1 Drop of Melissa Oil

Directions:

Mix all your ingredients together and apply as needed.

5. Mood Balancer Blend Diffuser Recipe

4 Drops of Clary Sage Oil

4 Drops of Neroli Oil

2 Drops of Jasmine Oil

Directions:

Add these oils to your diffuser and enjoy.

6. Focused Relief Diffuser Recipe

7 Drops of Cypress Oil

5 Drops of Lavender Oil

3 Drops of Grapefruit Oil

2 Drops of Vetiver Oil

2 Drops of Cedar Oil

Directions:

Add these oils to your diffuser and enjoy.

7. Rested Rejuvenation Blend Recipe

15 ML of Jojoba / Rose Hip Oil Blend

8 Drops of Clary Sage Oil

8 Drops of Vetiver Oil

8 Drops of Lavender Oil

Directions:

Mix all your ingredients together and apply as needed.

8. Gain Focus Diffuser Recipe

2 Drops of Peppermint Oil

2 Drops of Wild Orange Oil

Directions:

Add these oils to your diffuser and enjoy.

9. Rested Meditation Blend Recipe

30 ML of Jojoba Oil

8 Drops of Frankincense Oil

6 Drops of Sandalwood Oil

3 Drops of Cedarwood Oil

3 Drops of Frankincense Myrrh Oil

Directions:

Mix all your ingredients together and apply as needed.

10. Insomnia Relief Recipe

30 ML of Sweet Almond Oil

10 Drops of Roman Chamomile Oil

5 Drops of Lavender Oil

3 Drops Of Patchouli Oil

2 Drops of Cedarwood Oil

Directions:

Mix all your ingredients together in a dark bottle. Shake well. Massage mixture into skin thoroughly approximately 1 hour before bed.

11. Breathe Deeply Diffuser Recipe

1 Drop of Ylang Ylang Oil

1 Drop Of Patchouli Oil

1 Drop of Bergamot Oil

Directions:

Add these oils to your diffuser and enjoy.

12. Self Acceptance Recipe

5 Drops of Jasmine Oil

1 Blank Inhaler

Directions:

Place oil into your inhaler. Inhale deeply as needed.

13. Higher Self Confidence Recipe

3 Drops of Spearmint Oil

1 Blank Inhaler

Directions:

Place oil into your inhaler. Inhale deeply as needed.

Essential Oils Romance, Love, & Relationship Recipes

In this section, I'm going to give you some recipes that are perfect when you want to fan the flames of romance and love.

1. Feeling Wonderful Diffuser Recipe

15 Drops of Rose Absolute Oil

1 Drop of Geranium Oil

Directions:

Add these oils to your diffuser and enjoy.

2. Feeling Sweet Diffuser Recipe

2 Drops of Chamomile Oil

2 Drops of Ylang Ylang Oil

Directions:

Add these oils to your diffuser and enjoy.

3. Love Is Here Diffuser Recipe

5 Drops of Geranium Oil

3 Drops of Jasmine Absolute Oil

1 Drop of Patchouli Oil

Directions:

Add these oils to your diffuser and enjoy.

4. Romance Blend Recipe

15 ML of Marula Oil

4 Drops of Sandalwood Oil

4 Drops of Jasmine Oil

2 Drops of Cardamom Oil

2 Drops of Rose Oil

Directions:

Mix all your ingredients together and apply topically.

5. Sweet Cinnamon Diffuser Recipe

6 Drops of Tangerine Oil

4 Drops of Cinnamon Cassia Oil

2 Drops of Nutmeg Oil

Directions:

Add these oils to your diffuser and enjoy.

6. Romantic Nectar Love Potion Recipe

55 Drops of Orange Oil

41 Drops of Mandarin Oil

19 Drops of Sandalwood Oil

13 Drops of Vanilla Absolute Oil

11 Drops of Cardamom Oil

8 Drops of Ginger Oil

8 Drops of White Ginger Lily

7 Drops of Jasmine Absolute Oil

4 Drops of Patchouli Oil

Directions:

Mix all your ingredients together and apply topically. Avoid exposure to direct sunlight after application.

7. Smooth Love Potion Recipe

36 Drops of Ylang Ylang Oil

30 Drops of Rose Geranium Oil

15 Drops of Melissa Oil

13 Drops of Rose Absolute Oil

11 Drops of Ginger Oil

10 Drops of Zdravetz Oil

5 Drops of Cinnamon Oil

Directions:

Mix all your ingredients together and apply topically. Avoid exposure to direct sunlight after application.

8. Love Potion Blend Recipe

40 Drops of Sandalwood Oil

31 Drops of Vanilla Absolute Oil

20 Drops of Orange Oil

18 Drops of Neroli Oil

16 Drops of Mandarin Oil

12 Drops of Jasmine Oil

11 Drops of Cardamom

11 Drops of Grapefruit Oil

10 Drops of Saffron Attar Oil

8 Drops of Vetiver Oil

8 Drops of Blue Lotus Oil

8 Drops of Fir Oil

4 Drops of Marigold Oil

Directions:

Mix all your ingredients together and apply topically. Avoid exposure to direct sunlight after application.

Essential Oils Recipes For Your Pets

In this section, I'm going to give you some recipes that are great for treating your pets. I hope they help you as much as they have me over the years. Remember to always do your research on an oil before using it on your pets or yourself. Don't put the safety of your pet at risk because you didn't take the time beforehand to do your due diligence. Using essential oils on your pet inappropriately could lead to side effects including death.

1. Tick Repellent Remedy Recipe

60 Drops of Olive Oil

1 Drop of Lavender Oil

Directions:

Mix your ingredients together. Pour a couple drops on the tick and allow it to sit for a little bit. Extract the tick and wipe away any excess oil.

2. Skin Allergy Recipe

20 ML of Sweet Almond Oil

10 Drops of Lavender Oil

6 Drops of Chamomile Oil

5 Drops of Geranium Oil

2 Drops of Carrot Seed Oil

Directions:

Mix all your ingredients together. Rub 4 drops between your hands and apply to your pet's ears, between their thighs, and under their armpits.

3. Defeat Motion Sickness Recipe

20 ML of Jojoba Oil

12 Drops of Peppermint Oil

8 Drops of Ginger Oil

Directions:

Mix your ingredients together. Apply mixture to your pet's ears, thighs, coat, and armpits.

4. Combat Rheum Recipe

2 Drops of Eucalyptus Oil

Hot Water

Directions:

Mix your ingredients together. Allow your pet breathe in the steam. Be sure to keep your pet from burning themselves on the water.

5. Repel Mosquitoes Recipe

10 Ounces of Aloe Vera Juice

30 Drops of Citronella Oil

12 Drops of Myrrh Oil

12 Drops of Rose Geranium Oil

12 Drops of Lemongrass Oil

Directions:

Mix your ingredients together in a spray bottle. Spray over your pet's coat. Avoid the eyes.

6. Reduce Anxiety Recipe

20 ML of Sweet Almond Oil

8 Drops of Petitgrain Oil

6 Drops of Bergamot Oil

2 Drops of Ylang Ylang Oil

2 Drops of Sweet Basil Oil

1 Drop of Neroli Oil

Directions:

Mix your ingredients together. Massage a small amount onto the chest of your pet as needed.

7. Fresh Smelling Breath Recipe

20 ML of Sweet Almond Oil

10 Drops of Cardamom Oil

8 Drops of Coriander Seed Oil

6 Drops of Peppermint Oil

Directions:

Mix your ingredients together in a small sized glass bottle. Use a dropper and give your pets 3 drops every day to improve their breath.

8. Nice Coat Remedy Recipe

4 Drops of Rosemary Oil

2 Drops of Grapefruit Seed Oil

All Natural Shampoo

Directions:

Mix your ingredients together. Apply shampoo to pet and wash them with water.

9. Dry Paws Recipe

70 Drops of Coconut Oil

1 Drop of Lavender Oil

Directions:

Mix your ingredients together. Place on your pet's pads using a cotton pad. Can also put in special socks to keep them from getting at the mixture.

10. Arthritis Remedy Recipe

15 ML of Jojoba Oil

6 Drops of Rosemary Oil

4 Drops of Ginger Oil

3 Drops of Lavender Oil

Directions:

Mix your ingredients together. Massage mixture onto your pet's sore joints.

Conclusion

Thanks for checking out my book. I hope this guide on essential oils has given you a nice introduction to everything you need to get up and running. Don't wait on getting started. The quicker you begin, the quicker you'll start to notice an improvement in your well-being and overall health.

Not every essential oil is created equally. Choose the highest quality essential oils you can afford. Follow all the directions and safety precautions. Pay extra attention when using these items on pets, pregnant women, and children. It might take some time to build up a wide collection of essential oils but you'll eventually figure out what kinds of essential oils you enjoy and want to use on a consistent basis.

I hope you've liked all the different essential oil recipes I've included in this guide. There's an endless amount of recipes to try. Experiment and create your own once you've gained some experience. Stick to these recipes while you're still learning and developing your knowledge base.

Best of luck. I wish you nothing but good fortune!

www.ingramcontent.com/pod-product-compliance
Lightning Source LLC
Chambersburg PA
CBHW071352280526
45787CB00001B/294